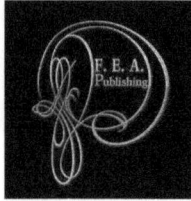

Published by F.E.A. Publishing, P.O. Box 438 St. Clair Shores, MI 48080. (586) 863-7636. First edition.

ISBN Number: 978-0-615-20180-1

Visit our website at: www.thistimesacharm.com
for more information about this book and the author.

Edited by Mike Valentino.
135 Beach Road, Unit C-3, Salisbury, MA 01952
Phone # 978-462-3013
editormikev@aol.com

Cover Design by Donald & Amy Wilhelm.
Cover Photo Credit: Scott Linsdeau
Website Design & Development by Active Media Architects &
Austin McLaughlin. www.activema.com

Visit www.booksurge.com to order additional copies.

THIS TIME'S A CHARM

Lessons of a Four-Time Cancer Survivor

Donald A. Wilhelm

Acknowledgments

To my wife Amy, thank you for your unquestioning support throughout this project. You never once doubted that we would make this book a reality and for that I am grateful. This is truly <u>our</u> book. I thank the Universe each day for you. I love you.

To my family who supported me and prayed for me throughout my years with cancer, I couldn't have done it without you.

To Dr. Jeffrey Margolis, we've been through a lot together and I appreciate all you've done for me. I'm positive that I'm not the easiest patient you've dealt with. Your tolerance of my requests and directives has been critical to our mutual success.

To my "East Side" friends, thank you for your well wishes and the laughs we've shared. And most importantly, thank you for not changing the way you acted around me just because I was going through treatments.

AUTHOR'S NOTE

This is my recollection of a certain 5-year period of my life. Wherever possible, names, events and characteristics have remained true to life. However, some names are fictitious and certain events may have actually occurred differently than I remember. Overall, not bad considering the periods of altered consciousness I've been through. :)

CHAPTER 1
Diagnosis

I had always hated doctors' offices, but on this Monday morning I would finally be given the justification for those old feelings. After six months of unsuccessful treatment by my family practitioner, I had been referred to an ENT (Ear, Nose and Throat specialist) for a persistent sinus infection. I was sitting on the exam table in an unusually posh exam room. I figured that someone had to pay for this nice office space. *That someone is about to be me*, I laughed to myself. The surgeon was across the room at the counter dictating some notes into my chart. She seemed happy after satisfying herself that I was an excellent candidate for her surgical services.

Just then, for no reason known to me, I felt the side of my neck.

"What do you make of these bumps," I asked.

She whirled around and hit the stop button on her tape recorder. The clicking sound was too loud, too deliberate. The doctor approached me immediately, almost running. She had a look on her face like I was now the dead, still talking. As she felt the nodules on the side of my neck, her mood turned somber in a way that made me feel completely alone. I was so scared that I sat there not registering my own existence. After what seemed like 7 hours, but in reality was only 7 seconds, she said, "You're gonna need to have biopsy surgery tomorrow morning. We need to rule out lymphoma."

In my head, I heard a screeching needle sliding across an old, vinyl record and it drowned out her last words to me. "I'm sorry, did... you just say I have... **CANCER!?**"

I'm not sure how I managed to make the 45-minute drive home because I had no recollection of the trip. No stop lights, no traffic, no speed limits, and no pedestrians. As I sat my wife, Sara, down on the couch I could see immense fear in her normally jovial green eyes. I bluntly spit out the news so as not to prolong her suffering. "I have to have a biopsy done in the morning. She thinks I might have cancer."

Sara paused for merely a second, leaned into me and we hugged like never before. She held me so tight to her chest that I had to breathe opposite of her just to have room to inhale and exhale. I was amazed by how quickly she rebounded from the news. At least on the outside. She straightened up, manufactured a smile and said, "Well, we don't know anything yet. Let's wait till we know for sure what it is. It might be nothing." I agreed with her …in principle, but I was a long way from all right.

If you've never had surgery before, you will learn that it is a much-disciplined chaos. The pre-surgery instruction phone call is very clear. "You are scheduled for surgery at 9 a.m. Nothing to eat or drink after midnight the night before. Be at registration by 7 a.m. Wear comfortable clothing." You know why they want you to wear comfortable clothing? Cause you're gonna be sittin' around and doin' a whole lot of waitin'. It's a closely held secret that the more surgeries that are scheduled before you, the more the Operating Room is behind schedule. If you happen to be unlucky and get a 1 p.m. surgery time, you better bring two books. In every surgical waiting room there needs to be a sign that reads: "Expect this to take longer than you're expecting, even if you're expecting it to take longer than you expect."

Around 10:30 a.m. the pre-op nurses finally started wheeling me down the labyrinth of hallways to the O.R. Once inside, the staff moved with the precision of Jeff Gordon's pit crew. I was quickly transferred from my gurney to center stage on the O.R. table. Two things struck me that I can never forget. 1) How unbelievably cold it is in an O.R. 2) How incredibly comforting the microwaved blankets that the nurses cover you with feel.

As show time approached, the anesthesiologist made some lame joke that the nurses laughed at out of trained obligation. He took pride in their coerced laughter. Not being able to shut off my quick wit, even in this situation, I one-upped him and caused a spontaneous roar in the O.R. Clearly wounded by my instant popularity, he leaned into me and began to push the anesthesia medication into my IV. He smiled a shit-eating grin of victory as he played his trump card. "Keep your day job," he whispered, and everything went black.

One of the observations that I made throughout my days as a cancer patient is that most people have no idea how to treat you when they hear you have cancer. I think that they must assume you're dying and that makes them very uncomfortable. They're probably struggling with their own mortality. They fidget and look away as they talk to you. They offer their heart felt sympathy but you can tell in their head they're saying things like, "Did that sound sincere enough? I hope he can't tell how uncomfortable I am. Why didn't anyone warn me about this before I ran into him? My God I hope he changes the topic soon."

What's even more noticeable than people's uncomfortablness with cancer is that most people have questions they want to ask, but they are afraid to, so they don't. It's like they think that you may be embarrassed about your disease and they shouldn't ask what they really want to know.

And without a doubt, there is one thing that people you run into, who know you have cancer, do more often than anything else. They lean in towards you, put their hand on your arm or shoulder, and say in a very slow and deliberate manner, "How…**arrrrrre**…you?" I now just have my own fun with them. My favorite response is, "Well, would you like the small-talk answer or the whole-truth-so-help-me-God one?" Then I quickly follow that up with a big reassuring smile and a, "I'm fine, thank you. How are you?"

After about a week, my biopsy results were complete. I did in fact have cancer, Hodgkin's Lymphoma. Hodgkin's disease is one of a group of cancers called lymphomas. Lymphoma is a general term for cancers that develop in the lymphatic system. Hodgkin's disease accounts for less than 1 percent of all cases of cancer in this country, although it's the most curable. It has a first time cure rate of approximately 86%. But if you know someone with Hodgkin's, please don't say anything like, "Well, if you're going to get cancer, that's the one you want, I guess." Though the intent of the statement is obviously to comfort, the words ring hollow. Cancer is not something that anyone wants in any form. Believe me.

I think some part of me knew I had cancer for quite some time. For six months I had been having night sweats, fatigue, sweating when I drank caffeine and a transient rash on my throat and eyelids. In fact, I took a printout from Web-

MD to my original family practitioner that listed eight symptoms of Hodgkin's. I told her that I had six of them. I tried to explain the mysterious rash but she belittled and dismissed me by saying, "You don't have cancer. What happens sometimes when you shave is that you get in-grown hairs that can cause a rash." She was already busy writing a script for an ointment. What?! "Doctor, you're not listening to me!! I don't shave my eyelids!!!"

That was the last time I ever spoke to her. In fact, I later tried to sue her for Failure to Diagnose, since she missed my cancer for six months and allowed it to advance to stage 4A, the second worst stage. I didn't want money; I wanted her to lose her license. But the attorneys that reviewed my case told me that we couldn't sue because she never put any of our conversations in my file. It would be my word against hers. How messed up is that? At best she's sloppy with her documentation and at worst purposefully negligent for not putting any of our conversations in my chart. And because of that fact, she is considered above reproach. Nice system.

CHAPTER 2
Choosing My Wagon Master

OK, now that I knew I had cancer, where would I go from here? It was immediately apparent that Sara and I were cut from the same cloth. We both instantly threw ourselves into researching everything about the disease. We devoured data about treatment options, survival rates, complementary nutritional regiments, faith healers, patient success stories and meditation. Within two days I felt I had been able to retain about 75% of what I need to know about my disease. I have always had a tremendous ability to learn new things quickly, if they were of interest to me. I believe I was blessed with an above-average IQ. In fact, both of my older brothers are members of Mensa, though I never bothered to be tested. I guess some part of me doesn't care to be judged and the other part doesn't want to be disappointed. And perhaps a third part that's just too lazy to take the test.

At the point I felt I was comfortable with my knowledge level regarding Hodgkin's, I set out to find an oncologist who would lead me through this terrible ordeal. From my experience with my family practitioner I had learned that not all doctors are good. It takes much more than medical knowledge to be a good physician. It takes empathy, good listening skills and an ego-check that says, "Hey, this isn't about me or what I know. This is about my patient and what he needs right now." I was searching for a doctor who could be comfortable with the fact that I was going to be calling the shots. His job would be to give me all of the information available, make his own recommendations and then respect my decision on the course of action. I knew that that wasn't going to be an easy search. I asked the ENT for a referral since she seemed to be plugged into a pretty good network of specialists. She gave me two recommendations. One guy worked at the University of Michigan. He was a savant when it came to oncology, but she said he had a pretty significant case of "White Coat Disease." Also referred to as the "God Complex," these are physicians who believe they know everything and the patient knows nothing. 'If you want to survive, you will do exactly as I say, with no questions.' I told her I would call him, but I was doubtful that I could work with someone like that.

She continued, "There's another young doctor at Beaumont. He just came from Johns Hopkins and I am hearing some great things about him." I told her I would start with these two recommendations and let her know where I ended up.

I scheduled an appointment with the University of Michigan's oncology department. Unfortunately, the physician I was referred to was far too brash, pompous and condescending for me. We didn't see eye-to-eye, and I had no intention of letting him be my wagon master. I was thankful for some information he gave me and overall he's a fine oncologist, just not the dedicated team player I was searching for.

So I moved on to the young doctor at Beaumont. I scheduled an appointment on a Wednesday to go for an initial evaluation. On Wednesdays, I found out, he's at another hospital, Botsford General. Sara and I packed up all of our research material and headed to our appointment. When we arrived, I was struck by how small and crowded the waiting room was. It was very uncomfortable because cancer patients are often in wheelchairs, so what started as a small waiting room felt more like a sitting area in the middle of a courteous bumper-car match. When they finally called us to the exam room, I heard some yelling coming from the treatment area. I took a peek back there. It was an even smaller room, with industrial armchairs lined up around the four walls. It was full of sickly looking, elderly patients who wore their diseases on their faces. As I walked back to my exam room, I heard one older gentleman pounding something on the wall begging for help from the nurses. He needed a bucket quickly because he was about to vomit. He pounded, in my opinion, for way too long before someone came for him. I went back into my room, looked at Sara and said, "There's no freaking way that I am getting treated by this guy! We'll stay to talk with him for the education, but then we're getting' the hell out of here. This place is a dump!" She had been thinking the same thing and was struggling with how to tell me.

After about five minutes, a young looking-oncologist named Dr. Jeffrey Margolis strolled into the room with a big smile on his face. It really struck me as unusual. Most people in his profession were somber a majority of the time. I would have thought that time would wear down a happy person, but he was seemingly unscathed. He went through the biopsy results with us, gave us more data to consider and recommended a treatment option. I let him talk for about 20 minutes. But I was still firm in my decision that I wouldn't be treated like the chemo cattle I had just seen in the other room. I had brought an obscure and very interesting study that I found during my research that came from The University of South Florida. I knew that physicians often used radiation in combination with chemo in treating newly diagnosed Hodgkin's patients. I also knew that radiation scared the crap out of me. I had pictures of Hiroshima victims running through my head at each mention of the word. The study basically showed that including radiation, though increasing the initial remission rates, had no statistically significant impact on actual long-term survival rates, due to the increase in potential for secondary cancers. I asked Dr. Margolis a question, as a trap to help justify my decision not to have him treat me. "I am very interested and optimistic in the research around combination therapy. Would you recommend radiation for me?" Clutching the study in my hands, secure knowing that he couldn't see what I was holding, I reveled in my perfect trap. "Actually," he said, "there's a new study out from the University of South Florida….wha wha wha wha…" His words droned on like Charlie Brown's teacher. I didn't need to hear anymore. I knew what he was saying and I had suddenly discovered a tremendous amount of respect for him.

We continued to talk, asking questions and posing what-if's. After 45 minutes of sitting with us, he leaned in and said, "Do you have any more questions for me?" Sara and I looked at each other, smiled because we both knew this was our new oncologist, and told him that we didn't. And then he did something that no other doctor has ever done in the history of the world, I'm certain of it. He sat back in his chair and said, "I'm sure that this has all been very overwhelming to both of you. I want to make sure you are totally comfortable with me. I'm going to sit here quietly for five minutes and wait to see if you come up with any more questions." In this day and age of managed care, decreased reimbursement rates and 80 hour work weeks, this is unheard of! We were totally hooked. We sat there for the full five minutes silent and uncomfortable. But the gesture had left an indelible impression on both of us.

"Where do we start, Dr. Margolis," I asked. He told me that I'd need to be staged, which involved some initial base-line tests and a bone marrow biopsy. He told me that I would have treatment for 2-4 hours once every other week. "What day would you like to have as your treatment day?" I was a little surprised that I got to choose. I chose Friday, wanting to be able to recover during the weekends for the smallest impact to my work schedule, since I had just started with a new company a month before. He said, "Great. I'm in my Beaumont office on Friday's. I think you'll find it to be much nicer than this place. Faux wood floors and a huge treatment area with leather recliners. By the way, since I work in a practice with my father and brother, a total of three Dr. Margolis', everyone just calls me Dr. Jeff. Keeps the confusion to a minimum." He was still smiling. I was really starting to like this guy when something came out of his mouth that bowled me over. He stood up to shake my hand as we were leaving, looked me in the eye and said, "I'm going to cure you. I want you to know that."

"That's what I'm paying you for," I said, simply trying to mask my shock from his statement.

CHAPTER 3
My First Bone Marrow Biopsy

The worst thing you can do before you have a bone marrow biopsy is read about other people's experiences with them. Some things are best to go into blindly. But I know some of you are like me. You need to know what to expect beforehand. For those of us who'd feel like streakers in church if we went into a new situation without knowing what we don't know, read on. The rest of you, skip this section. It will be for your own good.

Bone marrow biopsies are done as a "simple" outpatient procedure, usually in a semi-private hospital room. I put quotes around the word "simple" because there aren't any characters in the English language that mean, "He's being sarcastic as hell." For your procedure, they'll probably put you in a room that already has another patient in it. I found this awkward because this is a very traumatic and painful procedure. I really didn't like having a guy on the other side of a curtain listening in on my suffering.

Because I had done all of my research on biopsies, and knew that this was going to be the worst pain I would ever experience, I had standing orders with Dr. Jeff that I was to be given every drug imaginable. So before he got there, the nurses had started my IV and given me a lovely cocktail of Lorcet, Morphine and Ativan. All are supposed pain relievers and each have a slightly amnesic effect.

The door opened and in walks Dr. Jeff, smiling as always…with five residents in tote, two of which were females. I asked, "Aaaah…, are they showing a movie in here later, Dr. Jeff?" He laughed and said, "This is a teaching hospital and these are my 1st year residents. You don't mind if they observe the procedure, do you?" Well, given that I was now on the spot in front of six people and my IV cocktail had made me happily woozy, I agreed. Actually I don't think I agreed as much as I just didn't say what I really wanted to. *Yeah, that's cool. I want all these people, especially the chicks, to check out my white ass while you're torturing me. In fact, shouldn't we be waiting for Oprah's television crew?*

Dr. Jeff then informed me that his 4th year resident, Dr. So & So, would be performing the procedure, under his supervision. *Man, this just keeps gettin' better,* I thought. They had me roll over onto my left side, facing the wall. Sara had just enough room to squeeze in between the bed and the wall to hold my hand. Dr. So & So started by numbing the area of my hip bone, just above my right butt cheek. This is just local anesthetic, so it only numbs the skin and tissue immediately below. Come to find out later, there is no way to numb the bone or the marrow inside.

After a minute or so, he said, "OK, let's get this started." He practically climbed into the bed with me, grabbing my right hip with his left hand. I could tell by the amount of pressure he was using, he was holding on for something that I wasn't gonna like. I couldn't feel the needle enter my skin at all. I was starting to relax a little, thinking that all the people I read about online must not have been as smart as me. They must not have insisted on all the drugs. Still, I was concerned by the amount of pressure his left hand was putting on me. He was pressing into my hip with a lot of force, but he kept making disappointed groans and then the pressure would stop. Dr. Jeff said, "He's young, Dr. So & So. His bones aren't brittle like the older patients. You need to put all your weight into it." With that, Dr. So & So gave the needle a mighty shove and leaned into it like he was trying to push his girlfriend's Mazda out of a snow bank. I heard a pop just a split second before I felt the pain. The needle had finally pierced my bone. It was such an intense pain; I imagined that this is what it feels like to be shot. The bright side was it was a very short, fleeting pain. If that was the worst of it, I would live through this after all.

Unfortunately, the real pain is when they aspirate the bone marrow from inside the bone. Said differently, it hurts like Holy Hell when they suck the marrow out! Marrow is a mostly fatty substance found in the center of bones. It is highly concentrated with nerve cells and pain receptors. As the doctor began to draw the marrow into the needle, my entire body cramped instantly. It was as if I had a charlie horse from head to toe. I was in so much pain, a deep pain, that all I could do was cramp up and let out a yelp like a wounded dog.

Just then, I heard Dr. Jeff say, "Sara, are you all right?" Apparently there was a lot of blood from the entrance site and it was spraying all over Dr. So & So. My poor wife was crying and about to pass out, not from the site of my blood, but from the agony of seeing her husband suffering to such an immense degree. As

I squeezed her hand and grabbed her arm she started to regain her composure. No drug in the world could ever kill the procedural pain I was experiencing. But the emotional pain from seeing my wife suffer completely masked what Dr. So & So was doing. After nearly a minute, he was done. Thank God it's over! Everything I read was right. This was the worst thing anyone could ever have done to themselves.

Believing we were done, I was mentally returning to my happy place beside my wife when Dr. Jeff says, "OK, now we just gotta turn you over and do the other side."

You gotta' be fuckin' kidding me, I thought. Actually, I thought that I thought it, but apparently the Ativan had coaxed me into saying it out loud. I could feel the uneasiness that my comment caused in the residents. One of the female residents, wearing a red turtleneck sweater underneath her white lab coat, tried her best to comfort me. She said, "It sucks now, but you'll never remember any of this because of the Lorcet we gave you. It has an amnesic effect."

I rolled over and told Sara she probably should leave the room. She wished she didn't want to go. I know she felt like she was abandoning me, but we both knew she couldn't stay. Still crying, she left the room, and I told them sternly, "Get this over with." Unfortunately, this wouldn't be the last time Sara would have to leave too early.

CHAPTER 4
The House that Stress Built

As if my cancer ordeal and new career weren't enough strain and stress on a newlywed couple, Sara and I had just begun building our first house together. It was going to be a big, beautiful house on two acres in the far suburbs of Detroit. Neither of us had ever owned a home, let alone had one built from the ground up.

In the beginning we had so much fun meeting with the builder and choosing cabinets, carpeting, fixtures, etc. We both thought having our house high on that hill would add an appropriate amount of snootiness to this sleepy little neighborhood.

Our builder said it should take him 5-6 months to complete our house. During our first visit Sara and I danced around the giant hole in the ground, poured with our soon-to-be basement walls. We snapped pictures joyfully. "Alright Don, now let me take one of you with our new hole," she said playfully.

But two months later, as we struggled up the 20-degree slope of a driveway on foot, our hole had lost all of its charm. "They haven't done a fucking thing since the last time we were here," I said in disgust. Still, since I had never built a house, I was hesitant to go off the deep end just yet. Sara, on the other hand, being a professional project manager was mad enough to spit nails.

I spent the next 30 minutes calming her down, promising to call the builder on our way home, just as soon as we had a good cellular signal. All the while I was thinking to myself, *I have a chemo appointment tomorrow. This is about the last shit I want to be dealing with today!*

CHAPTER 5
My First Chemo Appointment

It was Friday afternoon and Sara and I were just getting introduced to the staff at Dr. Jeff's Beaumont office. In the front office we met a wonderful woman named Marsella. She was a medium-skinned black woman with the slightest hint of freckles on her face. She reminded me of the strong mother type, but respected because she was always fair. She is Dr. Jeff's office manager and she runs a tight ship. But she takes an interest in everyone by name and if you need anything, she <u>will</u> take care of it.

Next we were taken back to the lab area. This is Leslie's domain. Leslie could start a clean IV on you the first time if you were galloping past her on a quarter horse. Above her desk she has a huge collage of pictures, but the one that always grabbed my attention was the one in the middle, with her and a rapper named Ice Cube. "Oh, that one? Yeah, that's me and Cube at a concert downtown," she said. Her eyes beamed with pride from the memories that photo conjured up for her.

Next, we met with Dr. Jeff in one of the plush exam rooms for a few minutes. He explained our path from here. He warned me that there was a 100% chance that the chemo drugs he was going to give me would make me lose my hair in 2-3 weeks. I looked at him, smiled and said, "No, I don't believe I'm going to let that happen, Dr. Jeff. I'm not going to lose my hair." He flashed a smile as if to say, *"I appreciate your fortitude, but don't tell me my business, son, you're gonna be as bald as a cue ball in no time."*

Lastly, he was trying to sell me on the benefits of having an infusaport put in my chest. I didn't know what it was, and I sure didn't like the sound of it. Dr. Jeff explained, "It's implanted under the skin and is completely free of maintenance. Then, when we draw blood or give chemo, we just poke a needle into it through your skin. Ports are intended to save your veins and make things easier. Chemo will eventually make your veins small, hard and difficult to get a needle into." Dr. Jeff is a great oncologist, but he is a terrible salesman. His pitch about having <u>another</u> surgery to partially avoid needle pokes left me less than enthused and I politely declined. There was a faint hint of disappointment on his face as he led us out of the exam room. This was the first time I had trumped his recommendation. Overall, he handled it well. He would grow to expect that from me. We would truly be partners in this adventure.

After our consultation, Sara and I were taken back to the treatment area. It had Pergo floors, a huge wall of windows and eight leather recliners all lined up in a big, gentle U-shape.

Here we were introduced to Teresa. Teresa owned you once you passed back into the treatment area and her only concern was for the welfare of her patients. In my experience, all women can multitask by nature. Very few men can. But Teresa had a gift for juggling 8 chemo patients, 14 family members, 32 different drugs and their doses, 3 callers on the phone, 2 drug reps and an intern who didn't know his role, all at once, for hours at a time. She was the shining example of what an oncology nurse should be. I have no idea what she made for a salary, but I know that if you asked Dr. Jeff's patients, we would have all agreed that doubling it on the spot would still not have given her what she was worth.

So I sat in my recliner, farthest on the right end of the U. There was another nurse helping Teresa out with some of the "easier" workload. She came to me and said, "OK, let's get an IV started on ya." At this point, I was still deathly afraid of needles and of anyone harboring one. I rolled up my sleeve, pretending to be brave, and started to sweat. After she tied off the tourniquet, she started to thwap my vein with her middle finger. *That's about enough of that shit,* I thought to myself. When she had adequately pissed off my vein, she grabbed the IV needle and jabbed it into my arm. *Mmmm, that stings! Why does she keep playing with it? Every time she moves it, it hurts more. Does this woman know I'm about to punch her in the head?* Barely even acknowledging me she says, "Oops, I blew that vein. We'll have to try another one." Flash forward, more burning pain and another blown vein, she tried a third time. "I'm not having any luck on you. We'll have to try the other arm," she says, almost blaming me. After her fifth failed attempt, I looked down and noticed that number 5 <u>AND</u> number 4 needles were both still in my arm. I started thinking that this woman was going to have to poke every vein in my body. I pictured an IV in the side of my neck. In an instant my entire shirt was soaked with sweat and darkness started to close in all around me. I was passing out! What a scary feeling that is. Luckily, she recognized this fact, probably because she's made so many of her patients do it. She went and got me a can of Coke to drink and we took a little break.

I said to her, "You know what? I'd like to talk with Dr. Jeff before we go any further." After a few minutes Dr. Jeff came by and I firmly told him, "I don't care what you have to do, but that woman is never to touch me again. Are we clear?" He said yes and disappeared to the lab.

I was now feeling nauseous from nearly passing out when Leslie came back. I guess I must have caused quite a ruckus around the office and I think I even had Leslie off her game. It's not that she had a problem getting a good IV started the first time. She didn't. The problem was she didn't remember to put the cap on the end of the IV line **before** sticking me with it. As soon as Leslie punctured my vein, blood went squirting out the other end, all over the place. And I mean all over. What a mess. But I didn't really care. The IV was in and that's all that mattered at this point.

Once Leslie got all the blood cleaned up, Dr. Jeff came back to see how I was doing. He could tell I had calmed down now and he thought it was time to add a little humor to the day. He gently grabbed my forearm, looked at Sara with his big smile and said, "You just bought yourself a port my friend." He tapped my arm and walked off. I would schedule the surgery for the following week.

Even with all my pre-research, I didn't really know what to expect during my first chemo treatment. I sat in my leather recliner as the head nurse, Teresa, ran back and forth and hung new bags onto my IV pole. First came a couple of different kinds of steroids, which supposedly prevent nausea. Next, followed three different IV bags filled with three different flavors of chemo, all in varying sizes. And finally, a giant syringe filled with a lovely, bright red chemo called Adrimaycin. This regiment is the gold standard for treating Hodgkin's the first time and it's referred to by the acronym for the four chemo drugs that the cocktail contains, ABVD.

At the time I thought I had successfully manufactured a true positive mental attitude (PMA) towards all of this. Over time though, I came to realize that

PMA starts with a spark, not an explosion, and it takes time and constant fanning to coax the internal fire to a therapeutic level. And there's a much more important factor to account for before you bother to build that fire…you must truly remove **FEAR** from the mental campsite. Fear is a wheelbarrow full of wet sand that will extinguish the best-intended blazes in your heart.

After four hours of treatment, I was done. Teresa removed the IV from my arm and had me stand up. She pulled me in and gave me a back-cracking hug. Although I had just met her, we had grown very close, given the traumatic circumstances. "We always hug hello and goodbye in my area, Don." This seemed right to me.

We were on our way home, driving along I-696 West in Detroit, when it really hit me that I just finished my first chemotherapy treatment. I felt relieved, but still anxious about the days to come. *How would I feel tomorrow, or Sunday? Was my hair going to fall out? How many times would I throw up this weekend? How was I going to be able to do this for six months straight? What the hell is an infusa port anyway and what will that surgery be like next week?*

Sara and I got home that Friday evening and she got me all setup on the couch. TV remote in one hand, cold glass of water on the coaster, and plenty of vitamins, minerals and extracts to take. Within a couple of hours, I was actually getting quite hungry. We ordered pizza from Pizza Hut, and let me tell you, that was the best freaking pizza I've ever eaten. It would take me several months to put the pieces together, but it turns out for some reason on treatment day, all food tastes amazing to me. It's like nothing I've ever experienced before. So much so that I made it a tradition in later years that on treatment night all my friends and I would go out to dinner so I could experience food at its finest.

Friday evening came and went and the only side effects that I felt were difficulty falling and staying asleep. I would highly recommend that as you're leaving your oncologist's office with all of your prescriptions; have him/her throw in one for a sleep aid. You need something to counteract the anti-nausea steroids, which are known to keep people awake.

I woke up Saturday morning, barely having slept but feeling surprisingly refreshed. I still had both of my arms, both legs and my skin hadn't fallen off.

OK, maybe my imagination had run away from me just a little bit as I wondered what this first treatment would do to me. The first side effect I noticed didn't hit me until about noon that day. I started to feel really warm and flushed in the face. I went into the bathroom to take a look in the mirror. I was as red as a Macintosh apple. It looked like I had sat in the sun for five hours, wearing Crisco's SPF (-15) Negative 15. But this side effect was short-lived and was almost entirely gone within two hours. The day rolled on and I had been getting off the couch periodically, checking on what Sara was up to and puttsing around in the yard.

By the time dinner-time came, I was starving. I was soooo looking forward to eating again based on my experience the night before with the pizza. Sara and I cooked filet on the grill. As I cut into the perfectly juicy, medium rare piece of beef, my mouth was watering at an all-time high. I put the fork into my mouth, started chewing, and was appalled by what I tasted. The only way I can describe it is that the steak tasted "buttery and one dimensional." It's like there was some coating on my tongue that was mutating the taste of the steak. Tasted like someone had coated my tongue with butter and then dipped it into candle wax. Everything else I tried to eat had that same "buttery" overtone. What a disappointment! I then remembered some of the research I had done on the side effects of chemotherapy. One of them is called taste perversion. *Ah ha. That's what this must be.* In fact, the experts tell you not to eat your favorite foods after having chemo because you might just ruin your taste for them for the rest of your life. That "buttery" taste is palpable and mentally staining, even years later. Today, if I stop to think about it, I can still taste it in my mind.

Sunday, the only additional side effect I noticed was fatigue. I would start out the day feeling "OK," but come 1-2 p.m. I would hit a wall. I guess that's what football is for, eh?

Monday morning came, the alarm went off, I felt decent so I packed up my crap and went into the office. I hadn't had any vomiting all weekend, and really, overall I thought everything had gone very smoothly. It wasn't nearly as bad as I was told to expect. In fact, it was downright tolerable, although the steroids brought another little gift, constipation.

Overtime, I came to show all the people in my life that chemo doesn't have to keep you down. You need to know how to manage the side effects. You need to know when to take it easy, and when to tell yourself to get off your ass and go live your life. To sum up Dr. Phil, this isn't a dry run. Your life is right now, it's happening at this moment and no one is guaranteed any specific amount of time in this world. A guy that I worked with at the time uttered a phrase that has stuck with me to this very day. He was impressed with the fact that every Monday morning I'd be in the office, regardless of my treatment that previous Friday afternoon. He said, "I admire the way you're tackling this thing. One day at a time and you don't feel sorry for yourself. And you're not asking anyone else to feel sorry for you either. It's like you have an attitude that says, **it is what it is**." Those five little words collided with my psyche like a mid-sized Volvo, driven by the Insurance Institute's crash test dummies as they careen into the test wall at 55 mph. *It is what it is.* I still use that simple phrase in my everyday life. It has helped me cope with countless situations that would have otherwise taxed my patience or coping abilities.

As the months passed, I had become a favorite in Dr. Jeff's office. My positive attitude and quick wit were a pleasant change for the staff and even my fellow patients. As you can guess, most cancer patients are elderly. And it's rare to find someone with an upbeat attitude about chemo treatment. I have been asked so many times over my five years, "what are you doing in here? You're too young to have cancer."

I would reply, "I know. That's what I keep telling Dr. Jeff, but he insists that I have it all the same. I think he's just trying to make a buck."

My prankster side also got to shine in this environment. I remember one treatment day, they sat a young black man named Martin next to me. He was a newbie. He and I were talking before we got hooked up to our IV's and I was answering dozens of questions about what he should expect. He shared with me that he was deathly afraid of needles, and I reassured him that he'd get used to them. Little did I know that they had to give him a sedation pill while he was still in the exam room because of his anxiety over getting poked. I guess he literally had a panic attack. During our treatments that day, we continued to talk about family, work, vacations, and how cancer had affected us. At the end when Teresa came to unhook his IV I said, "Sweet. Looks like you're almost done. Congrats! All you have to do now is get that last injection into your tongue and you can go home."

As his brain processed my comment, the smile on his face crystallized, shattered into a million pieces and fell to the floor, leaving only a white outline of his features. I actually believe he was in the process of fainting when I bellowed, "Dude, I'm only kidding!! You're done! You can go home now." Everyone in the place erupted in laughter, and now relieved, he laughed right along with us. I had made a new chemo buddy right then and there. I'm not sure how many times Teresa has retold that story over the years, but Dr. Jeff said recently that it's still the office favorite.

One Friday, I was about to sit down in my recliner for my treatment when Dr. Jeff came over to me. He explained to me that he had a new patient starting chemo today and that she was very nervous. He said, "I don't want to pressure you in any way, but would you be comfortable talking with her and sharing your positive attitude?" I was truly flattered and agreed immediately.

I went into the room and Jenny and her husband were sitting apart in the exam room. She was sitting on the exam table, and he was in one of the three office chairs, about 15 feet away. Dr. Jeff introduced me and left the room, closing the door behind him. I said, "Jenny, can you do me a favor and go sit next to your husband in the chair over there?" She did, and I hopped up onto the exam table. There's something psychologically intimidating about having to sit on the exam table. It designates you as the one who's sick. The paper crinkles loudly when you sit and it announces to everyone that you're the one who needs saving. I wanted to remove her from the hot seat.

As I sat on the table, I summed up my experiences so far. I touched on the treatments, the side effects or lack thereof, and even about the supposed hair loss. I pointed out that it had been three months and I still had all of my hair!! I answered a few questions from both of them. I saw Jenny smile briefly and she breathed a sigh of relief. That in turn set her husband at ease. And it filled me with amazing warmth to be able to help them.

By this time, Dr. Jeff had returned to the room so I teased him about all the money I was spending on haircuts. He retorted, "Well, there have been a *couple* of documented cases where patients receiving ABVD didn't lose their hair."

I said, "Well Sir, looks like you've got to document one more." And of course, I had a "nanny-nanny-boo-boo" look on my face when I said it.

Over time, Dr. Jeff would have me talk with many of his first time patients, and I really enjoyed the feeling. In fact, the call to help others is a big part of what spurred me to write this book.

CHAPTER 6
My First Remission

My first six months of treatment were now over. Dr. Jeff ordered a CT scan and a PET scan to ensure that I was in fact in remission. A PET scan is a fairly cool technology where they inject radioactive sugar into your body, wait one hour for your cells to absorb it, and then send you through a special CT machine. Cancer cells absorb sugar at a rate that is up to five times higher than the normal cells around them. For this reason, a live cancer cell will gorge itself on the nuclear isotope-laced sugar and will "light up" on the PET results. The radiologist can then easily discern between active cancer cells and scar tissue, which is normally left behind after chemo treatment.

The results came in; my scans were clear. There was no cancer in me. Nada. Bubkiss. I was officially pronounced "in remission." My remaining commitment was to come in after 30 days for validation testing, and then once every three months for a year. That was a deal I was more than willing to sign up for.

Two of the scariest words I encountered during my dance with cancer were, 'in remission.' One would assume that the patient would be completely relieved to hear those words. The truth is you are. You're overwhelmed with joy. You swear off all your bad habits and you start out on your new life. Your entire perspective on life is permanently altered, almost always for the better. The sun feels warmer, the birds chirp louder, time with friends and loved-ones is more special. But what you don't detect is that a malignant fear is setting in. That fear will start in the very depths of your subconscious. It's a fear that the cancer will return. It's a fear that all the stories you've ever heard about folks losing their "battles" with cancer will eventually happen to you. *Why was I able to beat this monster and two people next to me died? If a million cancer cells can fit on the head of a pin, how can they possibly know that they got it all? If it does come back, what are my odds then, like 10%? What am I eating right this second? Pizza? That's not healthy!! My cancer could be growing back at this very moment!* Every little pain, every little crick in your body, every little bump under your skin, every little irregularity can send you into a negative mental spiral. *Oh my God, I've never had that feeling before. My cancer must be back!* It is injurious how often you begin to think about it returning.

In my case, I honestly could say that not 10 seconds went by any day that I didn't think about it and worry that my cancer was coming back. Can you imagine? If this anxiety is left unchecked, you will literally worry yourself to the point where your cancer will return. Believe me, I was my worst enemy when it came to the self-doubting statements I let my mind make.

Researchers have shown that anxiety, stress and worry all have a negative impact on your immune system. Chronic anxiety reduces the number of lymphocytes in the blood, or white blood cells, and also causes an abnormal release of corticosteroids from the adrenal cortex. These corticosteroids suppress the immune system from doing its normal functions. In fact, back in the early days of organ transplants, doctors would administer large doses of corticosteroids, post-transplant, to intentionally suppress the immune system and lessen the chance that the patient's body would reject the new organ. Clearly having all of my negative thoughts and anxiety was just setting me up for failure. It's easy to see now, but at the time it felt like a black hole pulling me into the dark.

Given anxiety's negative effect on one's immune system, I believe that every person who is diagnosed with cancer should be written a simultaneous referral to a psychologist who specializes in mental coping skills. Mental therapy should be the gold standard, prescribed concomitantly with chemo or radiation. Physicians will ask their new cancer patients to stop smoking immediately. That is because they know that smoking impairs the immune system. Why then, faced with the medical evidence that anxiety and stress have the exact, if not worse effect on the immune system, do doctors not send their new patients to a psychologist? How many minutes a day does a smoker smoke? Twenty cigarettes in a pack, two minutes to smoke each one. Forty minutes a day of injurious behavior. But in my case, I was spending 24 hours a day stressing about my illness. I'm sorry, but I don't care how tough you think you are. When you get diagnosed with cancer, you're gonna have a mother-load of anxiety! I believe so strongly in the mind/body connection that I think it's virtually malpractice for an oncologist not to make a psychological referral.

In fact, there's a whole new study in psychology dedicated to this concept called psycho-oncology. Psycho-oncology is the study of the psychological, social, behavioral, and ethical aspects of cancer. Psycho-oncology addresses the two major psychological dimensions of cancer: (1) the psychological responses of patients to cancer at all stages of the disease; and (2) the psychological, behavioral and social factors that may influence the disease process. It's still a pretty new area of medicine, but one that is receiving deserved attention. In an early study, more than 47% of cancer patients satisfied the *Diagnostic and Statistical Manual of Mental Disorders' (DSM)* criteria for mental disorder. Almost 1 out of 2 patients needed help with coping skills. I know I certainly qualified, and then some.

In any event, (climbing down from my soapbox long enough to continue the story) now that I was in remission, Sara and I returned to normal life. Enjoying my new title as a "survivor," I began to resume my everyday life. I honestly was eating better and taking better care of myself. I still never really dealt with the emotions from my cancer ordeal, but rather, I thought I had a spare closet in the basement of my subconscious that I could fit them into neatly.

After the 30-day post treatment mark, I went to my scheduled CT scan. As a veteran of this process now, I was in and out of there in one hour and change. I was looking forward to the vindicating results certain to follow.

Two days went by and I received a call from Dr. Jeff. "Don, I've reviewed the test results. All of your past spots look clear on the CT scans." His tone started upbeat and he had paused just long enough before his next sentence that my mind was halfway through a double back flip of joy.

"But there's a new area of white on the scan behind your forehead." I was silent. I wasn't breathing.

"I don't know what it is but Hodgkin's almost never makes its way into the brain."

The word "**ALMOST**" stood out in my mind as if it was typed in all caps, bolded, underlined and printed in a larger font than the rest of his words. I took a short breath as my mind went into overdrive. *Now I have brain cancer!!! Jesus Christ, who am I, Lance Armstrong? What are my odds now?* From my previ-

ous research I knew that malignant brain tumors were some of the fastest kill-
ers. My five-year survival rate would now drop from 86% to maybe 20%.

Dr. Jeff interrupted my internal panic, but even his words were burdened by
a tone of uncertainty.

"We need to schedule an MRI, test Don. It will show much more clearly what
this spot is on your brain."

In an instant, my emotions were plummeting to that dark place that I was so
familiar with by now.

If you've never had an MRI done before, I'll describe it to you. I had never had
one either and assumed it was similar to a CT or PET scan. Wrong. The MRI
machine is a long, narrow tube with a floating table that moves in and out of
it. You lay down on the table and it slides you into a very tight space in a very
big machine. It's a giant, electronic coffin. I'm not claustrophobic, but it was
very easy to imagine what it might feel like to be buried alive. The rounded
ceiling of the machine above me was just inches from the tip of my nose. I
could actually feel my breath reflecting off the ceiling above me. I found myself struggling to breathe until I calmed myself down.

The technician began the test by pushing the start button and it was under
way. There were many series of clicks and pops that the machine made as a
normal part of its process. But occasionally there was a loud "BANG" and it
absolutely scared the crap out of me! The test was so obtrusive that I didn't
think about the spot on my brain once. Testing went on for what seemed like
an hour. I was never so happy to be out of somewhere than I was from that life-
saving coffin. Per usual, I would have to wait 2-3 days for the test results.

A couple of days later, I had to go on a business trip to Cincinnati. For this
particular trip, my company rented a conversion van so all the employees,
seven of us, could ride down together. It was a jovial mood with many jokes
and rips flying around the van. We exited the freeway somewhere in Northern
Ohio to get gas for our rattle-trap-gunship. I remember just as we were pulling in, my phone rang. I knew the number… it was Dr. Jeff's office. My buddy
next to me saw my face drain of the group's jovial mood and turn to stone. He

had been around me during my diagnosis and treatments, so he knew who was on the other end of that call. I answered the phone.

"Mr. Wilhelm, this is Dr. Jeff's office calling. Can you hold for the doctor? He has some test results for you."

I felt my emotional foundation buckle. I had instant thoughts of doom. *My God, I really can't deal with brain cancer. I'm not over what just happened to me with the last round of treatments. You know what, I'm just going to accept my fate and give up...* Just then my negative nosedive was interrupted by Dr. Jeff's voice. He didn't even say hello. He's the kind of doctor that knows this is not an occasion for small talk. "It's just a sinus infection," he said laughingly. "I'll fax over an antibiotic prescription to your pharmacy this afternoon." I felt the warmth of my blood returning to my hands and feet. I felt the color flood back into my face. I felt the tightness in my chest and shoulders release. And as I hung up the phone, it's as if I was standing on the beach, facing the ocean and about to be hit by a tsunami wave. But this was a giant wave of happiness, joy and gratitude, and I yearned for its arrival. I deserved this wave.

Carrying my renewed gratitude with me, I threw myself back into my work. As a professional sales rep in the Information Technology field, days are long and nights are short. There's always another call to make or another deal to work on. I feel I have a mental skill that gives me an advantage over the rest of the field. I cannot stop my mind from playing, replaying and hypothesizing about scenarios surrounding the deals that I'm trying to win. Every conversation is replayed and my subconscious digs for another meaning or reference in the words. What this skill allows me to do is better position myself and product or service over my competition. I anticipate their moves and lay traps along their eventual route. It's a very involved chess game, and I really love it.

Traditionally with a sales career comes a ton of freedom. I work from home, and my manager is located four states away. I set my own schedule as I pursue my deals. Do I schedule any meetings at 4 p.m. on a Friday afternoon? Come on, do you even need me to answer that? But saddled to that freedom comes great responsibility and stress. No company survives long without new revenue and new customers. It is the success of the sales reps of the world that drive the bottom-line growth to fuel corporate expansions, pay raises, afford mergers and pay for new product development. The pressure to perform, especially in the I.T. field is overwhelming at times. A manager once told me, "Don't mistake efforts for results. I'm not here to baby sit you and I'm not asking you to *look* busy. I'm expecting you to make your quota. Period." The pressure in this job is absolute. This is the environment that I dove back into following my clean test results.

You know how millions of people make New Year's resolutions on January 1st, only to abandon them 30 days later? Studies of average Americans show that at least 50% have abandoned their resolutions by January 31st, and up to 90% by March 31st. As embarrassed as I am to admit this, I think "remission resolutions" last about the same length of time. I believe it's human nature to slip right back into your old habits and to become a product of the environment you spend most of your time in. When I was working 12 hours a day, along-side younger reps who are eating tacos, pizza and consuming mass quantities of alcohol each day, a well-intentioned resolution to eat more fish and workout five times per week gets lost in the shuffle.

I see now that my mistake was simply placing my priorities in the wrong place. I was defining success by how well I got along in life and how many material things I could accumulate. From the time I was a boy, my Mom would always refer to my older brother Joe's success. "You should be more like Joe," she would always say to me. Joe had gone straight to college with honors, began a career with Unilever Corporation, got married young, and had two kids; a boy and a girl. He worked his way up the corporate ladder over his long career and at present sits high atop the world as Chief Financial Officer of ConAgra's Food Division, which is approximately an $8 Billion per year business. What my Mom and I had failed to understand is that my brother Joe's definition of success is only one opinion. Thankfully for me, I would come to define success quite differently. I now realize that I like to get out and enjoy life in the present, while I can. I want to live life to its fullest. And most of all, I define success as being happy, plain and simple. Nothing else matters.

Chapter 7
Relapse #1

Flash forward three months. I had scheduled a meeting with a new potential customer. I had managed to get several of their Vice Presidents and a couple of other extremely important executives into this meeting. Recognizing the importance of this meeting, I had brought several members of my management team from out of town. The meeting progressed in the usual fashion. They explained their business and each of their roles within it. Then we explained our core competencies and how we could help them if only they'd spend some money with us. This 1-hour meeting had been going on for approximately 40 minutes and by any accounts was a huge success. I sat and listened to my manager speaking, "Well Gentlemen, given that we have 18 years of experience helping clients just like you with these exact issues, I'd like to suggest that …"

Just then I felt a strange twinge on the left side of my throat, down at the bottom where it meets my chest. The sensation was sharp, though it didn't really hurt. Responding with autonomic reflexes, I instantly put my left index finger on the exact spot where the sensation was coming from. In a heartbeat, I was a million miles away from that meeting. My life was parading past me, almost taunting me that I was no longer in control of it. Mentally, I felt beaten down. I was energy-less. Under my finger was a tumor. My cancer was back, and only a few months after I had gotten rid of it.

Following our meeting, my manager and I had lunch together. This was normal since he was from out of town and we liked to catch up on things with the limited time we could actually meet in person. Our waitress took our drink orders, he a Diet Coke and me an iced tea. After our drinks arrived, he said in his gentle West Virginian accent, "Don, what happened in that meeting today? Everything was going along great, and all of a sudden you simply disappeared. I noticed it kind of made everyone a little uncomfortable."

His questions were completely fair and well intended. But I hadn't had the chance yet to come to terms with my cancer's return. It seems, as with my original diagnosis, I needed about two hours to run the gamut of emotions within me, before my psyche could harden enough to support this added stress. I stammered my way through the explanation of what happened and did my best to answer his follow-up questions. "What does that mean for you, Don? What happens next?"

"I don't really know. I'm pretty sure my odds just dropped substantially... probably gonna need a bone marrow transplant...likely gonna have to go on long-term disability." His face filled with emotions, and it was clear he didn't know what to say. I put on as happy of a face as I could muster at that time and said, "I'm really not sure of anything at this point. Let me see my doctor and get more info. No matter what happens, I'm going to be fine."

Those words were meant for his peace of mind, not mine. To me, I was lying to him for his own good, because that's what good cancer patients have to do sometimes. We show strength for others to spare them the reality of the situation. It's the ultimate irony in my mind really. We are the ones with a life-threatening disease. But yet we tell friends and family a rosier version of the truth, in order for them to avoid the emotions that an accurate depiction would bring them.

Later that same afternoon I stopped by Dr. Jeff's office. He felt the nodule in my neck and ordered a battery of tests. All of which I knew were a waste of time and money. I was beginning to establish an open line of communication with my body. It had already told me what those results would say. All of the tests would confirm my body's hints. My cancer was back with a vengeance.

I drove home that afternoon, expecting to receive a similar response as last time from Sara. I would explain that my cancer had returned, she would be shocked and scared momentarily, and then she'd say something like, "You beat it last time and you'll have no problem doing it again."

But I couldn't have been more wrong if I tried. We were sitting in the living room, I on the purple-hued sofa that she had to have from Art Van Furniture, and she in the matching chair. As I started to break the news to her, a glimmer of my Positive Mental Attitude already reemerging, her face betrayed her. She was trying to listen and ask relevant questions, but her eyes looked at me as if to say, "You poor guy. Your timing couldn't have been worse." Sara stood up and began to pace between the living room and the open kitchen. She had something she needed to tell me and now she was struggling with telling me or putting it off some more. She performed trivial housekeeping duties as she paced, trying to keep her mind free of what her mouth was saying. "Don, I love you more than anything. I am so sorry this is happening all over again to you, because you of all people don't deserve it. But I simply can't bear watching you go through another round of treatment...not now. I'm still not over the first one, and it's back already." She moved a magazine from the kitchen island onto the coffee table next to the stone fireplace. "This hurts too much and it's going to break me." I sat silently, my heart cracking at the corners. As she slid the salt & pepper shakers two inches back into their normal resting place, she dropped the rest of her bomb. "I can't go on like this. We need some time apart. Very soon." With that she collapsed back into the chair and began crying belligerently. A short conversation ensued, me trying to understand, and her trying to explain. Neither of us did a very good job with it. I became very stoic and rigid. I was hurt so deep I can't describe it, even today. To me, this was the ultimate betrayal. Her timing couldn't have been more selfish. I wasn't angry, but just immensely sad. I knew this wasn't the type of person she truly was. I knew this was a result of poor communication in our relationship. I knew all of this could be fixed. But to call it quits now, after what I just told her? I still don't get it.

So the very next weekend, "we" had decided that I needed to leave our house. A house that I only got to enjoy living in for a short few months. Although she offered to leave, it didn't seem genuine and besides, it was not in my nature to let her. I called my cousin Dave. He owned a very nice 4-bedroom, 2.5 bath home near Waterford, Michigan. "Dave, you still live alone in your bachelor house with 3 open bedrooms, right? Without forcing me to explain this over the phone, how would you feel about a renter for a short period of time?"

Dave asked no questions, which must have been hard for him since he, like most of my friends and family, had really grown to like Sara. But sensing my complicated situation, he excitedly said yes to my inquiry. "How soon can you get here?"

He offered to help me move my belongings, which I readily took him up on. Dave is the kind of man that people often turn to when they need help. He's selfless, genuine and can always be counted on at every turn. To say that he's a rare breed these days is as obvious as the words on this page.

One of the first things that Dave said was meant to welcome me. He told me, "Just because my name is on the mortgage for this place, doesn't make it less of your home. You share the bills with me, so you should think of this as ½ your home." I truly appreciated the sentiment but moving out of my house and facing a divorce, it was extremely uncomfortable for me to live there. Even though we were the only two people living there, well except for his two cats, I felt overwhelmed by it all. It didn't feel like my home. I missed my wife. I missed my dog. I missed my health. I missed my house out in the country. I missed the plans that Sara and I had made. Even though Dave's house was 1800 square feet, I stayed in my small bedroom a lot. It took me nearly a month to start to feel comfortable there.

During that first month at Dave's, I was also meeting regularly with doctors to determine my path for treatment. Dr. Jeff was suggesting an Autologous Stem Cell Transplant. I took the information he gave me and told him I'd get in touch, after I did all of my required research. During the next two weeks, I ruthlessly scoured the Internet for anything I could find on the topic. I also received two second opinions, the first by a well respected gentleman out of the University of Michigan Hospital. The second one was from a world-renowned expert in Hodgkin's treatment at Stanford University, Dr. Sandra Horning. Both doctors concurred that what Dr. Jeff was suggesting was the best chance for me to survive my disease at this point. Given that three out of three experts agreed, I thought to myself, *it doesn't look like you're going to avoid it this time old boy. You better learn to love this route and that means a Positive Mental Attitude towards it!*

I went to Dr. Jeff to let him know my decision to have the transplant and to pick his brain a little about what to expect. He said, "Well first off, I'm writing you a prescription to give to your company and to your insurance company. You'll need to go onto disability for this treatment." This revelation was a serious call to reality for me. Dr. Jeff was done screwing around with this cancer. He was reaching into his toolbox and he was pulling out the biggest hammer he had.

He continued, "We'll start out by getting you a new kind of port implanted into your chest. It's another kind of intravenous catheter, but this one is external. Basically it looks like three different bendy straws coming out from the same spot in your chest. They all feed into a central line inside the chest that's connected to your heart. We'll give you a week of chemo and that will cause your body to produce a huge amount of stem cells. Then we'll collect and freeze them. When they collect your stem cells they'll need the extra lines. This lets them pull blood out of you, circulate it through a filtering machine, and put it back into you continuously."

Dr. Jeff explained that I would have to go to another hospital to have the transplant done because it required a specialized program that Beaumont Hospital didn't have at the time. I chose the Karmanos Cancer Institute in downtown Detroit because I had read some good things about them online and in the local papers. Dr. Jeff said he could do the first part of the program, known as a conditioning regiment. He had Marsella set up my surgery for my new bendy straw catheter for later that same week.

As I waited for my surgery, I continued my research on the Internet for anything I could find on the topic of autologous stem cell transplants. The more I read, the more I dread. I made a list of the possible side effects and taped them above my desk in my bedroom. It included: *increased susceptibility to infections and bleeding, severe exhaustion, inability to climb a single flight of stairs, severe acne, graying of the skin, nausea, diarrhea, vomiting, constipation, loss of appetite, mouth sores, thrush (yeast infection in the mouth), hair loss, skin reactions, infertility, cataracts, secondary cancers, liver damage, kidney damage, lung damage, heart damage, and death.* Oh please, I sarcastically joked to myself. *That's the best they can do? What about flaming urination, smacking of the funny bone and uncontrollable hiccups?*

CHAPTER 8
Hamilton Hotel

One evening after my many medical appointments, my cousin Dave and I were sitting around in his living room watching TV. Out of nowhere Dave's blurts, "Oh my Bro is moving in with us, he got a job up here at Chrysler." I was happy to hear this because I had always liked both Dave and his brother Kevin and I thought it would a good time. Then almost under his breath Dave says, "Oh, and his girlfriend is coming too....and she has two cats."

Humph, was my internal reaction. These living conditions seemed less comforting now with all the details. Just as I had started to feel like Dave's house was my new home, there are now two more people and two more cats moving in. I had no control over what was happening and that made me feel like a guest all over again. But I chose to appreciate the fact that Dave was helping them out, just like he helped me out. They needed him and he was coming through. *I'll just have to get used to it. It is what it is.*

CHAPTER 9
Stem Cell Transplant

The process of an autologous stem cell transplant is very interesting to me. First I need to give you a little background on what a stem cell is and does. The majority of stem cells are in your bone marrow. The blood also contains some. Bone marrow stem cells magically turn into white blood cells, red blood cells, or platelets depending on what your body needs most at the time. It's really quite amazing if you think about it.

The stem cell transplant process starts by receiving a week of conditioning regimen. This is five days of chemo treatments. The chemo shocks your system and kills off a lot of living blood cells. Your bone marrow realizes this and releases a flood of new stem cells into the blood to begin to replace the lost cells.

Following the conditioning regiment, they collect many of those new stem cells from the blood through a special machine. They then freeze them.

Next, they bombard your body with high dose chemotherapy for another five days while you enjoy your no-frills stay in a special ward at the hospital. The theory is that chemo should wipe out all the cancer, but unfortunately it also takes a lot of healthy immune cells down in the friendly fire. Essentially at this point you have no immune system.

They then inject your own stem cells back into you. Over a period of 1-3 weeks, those stem cells start to grow back into red blood cells, white blood cells or platelets. This process is known as engraftment.

From there your body rebuilds its immune system and the cancer should be wiped out from all the chemo.

That's the entire process in a nutshell. Of course there are a ton of little things that happen along the way. And there are even more complications and/or side effects that can and will crop up. I'll touch on all of those as we move forward in my own personal journey.

It was time to begin my transplant. The whole process gets kicked off with five days of continuous chemo in what they call a "conditioning regimen." With a name like that, you'd think it was something healthy, like diet and exercise, wouldn't you? Not even close. Every day, for five days, I went into Dr. Jeff's office and sat through 2-3 hours of chemotherapy. And when I left, they hooked me to a two-liter bag of another kind of chemo. That bag then went inside of a backpack and was continuously fed into my vein through a small pump. It would slowly pump the nasty mixture into me over the next 20 hours or so. Each day we'd repeat the process: chemo in his office, take the chemo backpack home overnight, come back to the office the following day for more chemo. Have you ever had to shower with a backpack hooked to you? Let me tell you something right now, it ain't easy. I found that the easiest way was to put it on a very heavy hanger like one of those wooden ones with the metal hooks. I then strung it over the shower rod, leaving the bag on the outside of the shower. The key here is to make sure you ask your doctor for plenty of slack in the IV line. You can always coil up the extra and tuck it into the backpack. Trust me here, you'll need to be able to put some distance in-between you and that bag at times.

I have to be completely honest with you at this point. Sometime during this week I had felt the worst sickness I had ever known. I was already on heavy doses of steroids to help fight the nausea and vomiting. I was so sick that I asked Dave to take a picture of me so that I could remember how badly I felt. I needed a record of it. Truly, I was amazed that I was able to manufacture a smile for the camera.

The third day of office chemo treatments was horrible. I was receiving my daily infusion and I told Teresa that I was stopping the treatment half way through.

"I can't do this anymore! I can't take it. This is killing me. I'm quitting so please cancel the transplant."

Well evidently this type of reaction was one that was known to Dr. Jeff and his staff. Dr. Jeff came over, not in a placating way but rather a relaxed and practiced one. He conveyed that he understood how badly I was feeling. I seriously doubted that he could possibly have know how I was feeling given that he'd never been on the receiving end of this "conditioning regimen." He made it clear, in no uncertain terms, he was not dismissing me from the transplant. He still had several other drugs to treat the nausea with. He said, "Don, you're stronger than that. There's a reason that I've been asking you to speak with my new patients when they come in for their first treatment. Your heart and spirit inspire them to get through this stuff. You can do this." Damn him. Maybe he was a better sales rep than I had given him credit for after all.

He was right. I had panicked when I reached what I thought was my summit of sickness. I really did have the strength and positive mental attitude to get me through this. That conversation proved to be invaluable to me as I went forward. It became my base camp of emotional stability and determination. I would learn soon that I had not yet reached my sickness summit. In fact, I was still in the parking lot, near the trailhead where the mountain climbers stage their gear prior to beginning their ascent.

After I finished my fifth day of the regiment Teresa unhooked my IV and said, "I'm done with you. Go home. Get better and don't forget to visit us after your transplant." It's difficult to describe the feeling of leaving the office without that damn bag hooked to me. I felt free, as if acquitted of false charges.

It's bad enough that you have to get five days of continuous chemo, but then throw public embarrassment on top. People just look at you funny when they see the IV line running out from the top of the bag and into your shirt. The public treats sick people differently. They keep a little extra distance between you and them. They speak a little slower. They whisper to their coworkers or friends.

When I got home that evening, Dave informed me that a friend of his from work was getting relocated to Germany for Chrysler. For a short time, she needed a place to stay so she didn't have to sign a new lease with her landlord and then abandon it when she moved overseas in <u>two</u> months. She AND her boyfriend AND her two cats would be moving in next week. Sounding familiar? This time, it didn't go over very well with me. *Is he fucking kidding me? In a matter of months I went from sharing a brand new 2400 square foot house with my wife, to living in an 1800 square foot house with 6 adults and 6 cats?!?* Since Dave's announcement sounded less like an invitation for my opinion, but rather a last minute press release, I bit my tongue. I took the opportunity to pity myself, since no one else seemed to. I was very upset that Dave would do that do me. *Can't he see how sick I am? Can't he put himself in my place? Hell no, I don't want to live in this situation! Who would?*

Overtime, I would realize that, though Dave is not the world's best communicator, he does have one of the biggest hearts. This friend at work had come to Dave and asked for help with her predicament. It would seem that Dave is often incapable of not helping people when they need it. He puts himself second, and helps friends and family in need, period. He is unwavering in his efforts to support. I couldn't stay mad at him long. Oh, I tried…believe me. ;)

A couple of days later I had a check-up appointment with Dr. Jeff. He asked how I was doing, knowing that I was dealing with this transplant while going through a divorce on the side. I lied with a straight face and played the good patient. I wasn't going to burden him with my issues, even though they likely were impeding my healing process. But I did take the time to share the "funny story" about my current living conditions. Dr. Jeff said in mild shock, "You're living in a house with six cats? Oh, that's no good! You can't be around them after your transplant. You will have ZERO immune system and will be susceptible to several diseases that cats carry which are normally harmless to adults." Dr. Jeff's tone began as my physician's. But by the time he finished, he sounded more like my father after I played with matches and caught the long grass under the old station wagon on fire. "You have to move out, and I mean immediately."

The next day I rented a one-bedroom apartment about 10 minutes away from Dave's house. Dave helped me move my stuff, of course. It turned out to be one of the best things that ever happened to me. It was the first time in my life I had ever lived alone and the timing would end up to be simply perfect.

Somewhere around three days after the conditioning regiment your bone marrow releases a wave of stem cells into the bloodstream. That's when the transplant really kicks into high gear. I went to a special lab inside of Karmanos. The lab tech had me lay down in one of three hospital beds. Next to each bed was a large machine that looked like a kidney dialysis machine. Or at least how they look on TV. Each bed had a little TV on an extending arm that you could swing over your abdomen and watch your favorite day-time shows. That added feature to the hospital bed should serve as a warning flag to you. I now know it means, "Sit down. Take a load off. Don't be in a hurry. You're going to be here a long time."

Once in the bed it was time for my new, bendie-straw catheter to do its part. The tech explained what I was about to experience as she ran through the steps for stem cell collection. "I'm hooking an IV line up to your catheter. That line then runs into this Apheresis machine. Your blood circulates through the machine and it collects just the stem cells. Then the blood runs out through this other line and back into your catheter. And don't worry, there's less than a pint of blood outside of your body at any point in time."

Well, to me that seemed pretty simple. I asked, "How long will this take?" The tech's smile showed a sign of weakness. "Well...that all depends. Some people have more stem cells present in their blood than others. We usually run the machine for 5-6 hours on the first visit." I felt the question erupt from my mouth before I could stop it. I blurted out, "**First visit?** How many times do I have to do this?!?" The smile on her face was now entirely gone. "Can't tell really. Some people have to come 4 or 5 days in a row to make sure we harvest enough cells for the transplant to be effective. I'm sorry."

Her entire face now stoic, she focused on the task at hand. She hooked my catheter up to the machine and pushed the start button. The wheels on the machine started to spin and a gentle whir followed. But almost as quickly as we started I could tell there was a problem. My blood wasn't flowing out of the catheter line. Nothing was coming out. The tech's face grew casually solemn. She said, "Looks like one of the lines is clogged. This happens once in a while. I'll inject some clot busting drugs into the line and we'll try it again in 30 minutes." After 45 minutes it was obvious that her salvage attempts were not going to work. She explained in an unsteady voice, "We're only going to be able to use your catheter for the return blood flow out of the machine. I'm going to have to put an IV line into your arm to draw the blood out of." *Sure glad I had that surgery to get this catheter implanted,"* I thought to myself.

As she surveyed my arm, I surveyed her face. She was trying to get an IV started in my chemo-ravaged veins. We settled on one in my left forearm because I had had good luck with it recently. Her eyebrows lifted and her eyes were as big as gobstoppers. Her face was as easy to read as a honey-do list placed under your favorite mug next to the coffee maker. Her face spoke to me, *I hate when I have to do this. 99% of the time I get to use the catheter. I hope this works.* In fact it did work...for about five minutes. Then the blood flow ceased again. This time she was more confident on how to solve the problem. She put a large saline bag into the microwave. "Funny time for an odd tasting tea," I joked. She laughed out loud, more from me shattering the tension than from any real humor on my part. "No, the needle gauge I have to use in your arm is very large in order to get enough volume of blood into the machine. Since your veins have had so much chemo already, they're not much larger in diameter than the needle. What happens is your vein starts to spasm, which causes it to close off and stops the blood flow." She lays the toasty bag of saline across the IV site. It felt wonderful. Shortly thereafter, the blood began flowing again. "The warmth stops the vein from spasming," concluding her lesson in *Old-School Tricks for Modern Day Healthcare.*

Finally, after 10 hours of heating and reheating the saline pack, I was at last released for the day. I was given instructions to call the lab at 7:30 tomorrow morning. They will have the test results from my blood collection. They would actually count the stem cells they collected to determine if we had enough. If not, I'd have to return to the machine the following day for more of the same.

A restless night behind me, I dialed the lab's phone number. "Let me pull your report, Mr. Wilhelm. I'll be right back." I was put on hold and a recording played. It glorified the Karmanos Institute for their use of cutting edge technologies and procedures. I think of the heated saline bag and chuckle. The human on the other end of the line comes back on. "OK, great news, Donald! We collected more than five times the normal amount of stem cells on the first visit. You don't need to come in anymore." Wahoooo! I was overjoyed and oddly proud of my ability to produce five times the normal amount of stem cells. I thought to myself, *At every turn, I'm going to do better than the normal person. I'm going to beat this thing this time around for sure!* This time though, something weird happened in my mind. When I made that statement, it was as though I was shouting into a huge ravine. But when it was time for my voice to echo back to me, the words had changed. It was my voice at triple-speed saying, *You're in trouble. You'll probably die.* This was the first instance that I noticed my negative voice inside.

Dr. Phil McGraw calls these negative thoughts "tapes" in his book *Self Matters, Creating Your Life From the Inside Out.* It happens at a subconscious level and so fast that we don't really "hear" them. For me, it's almost always negative, saying things to myself that I wouldn't expect from my worst enemies. I was appalled at what I was telling myself. But as time went on, I would learn that stopping the tapes is hard enough, let alone re-recording them with positive thoughts.

So there I was, lying on the sandy beach in Aruba. I was spending the day on the Marriott's private 40-acre island. The beach chairs were all lined up for the tourists' daily visits. I had come over on the first water taxi of the morning to beat the crowds and the heat. I was told that only one other crazy person was up that early and in fact had already been swimming. I rationalized to myself, *It's only crazy because you work in this place and have lost your appreciation of its beauty. And besides, it's already freaking 90 degrees here at 8 a.m. I need to be around the water.*

I relaxed and was concentrating on the warm rays from the sun as they began to climb over the man-made stone break wall at the edge of the lagoon. I could see someone down to my left doing the same. She was Caucasian. A beautiful blonde, very sexy, especially her long legs. Her right leg was accented by a shiny silver ankle bracelet. Since I was single and she was apparently alone, I grabbed my umbrella drink and started to walk over. She glanced at me and welcomed me further with a smile. I was still about 10 yards away from her, when from the beyond the break wall came a shrill, repetitious sound that stopped me in my tracks. The sound kept a perfect 2-count as I looked around trying to figure out what the hell it was. "Ehg..Ehg..Ehg..Ehg..Ehg.." I looked at the woman but she was paying no attention to the sound. *How could she not hear it? It's deafening!* And with that final glance, I sat up in my bed, disgusted by the realization that my alarm clock had just interrupted what could have been my most successful relationship in a long time.

As I regained my senses, the reason for the alarm being set in the first place came back to me. My stomach dropped and a shiver raced down my spine, eventually lodging in my midsection. I had to get in the shower right now. My transplant starts in an hour. I joked out loud, "I wonder what kind of umbrella drinks they'll have in the hospital."

My parents had come down from Northern Michigan for my transplant and my oldest brother Joe had flown in from Connecticut. I was glad they were there for support because I was feeling very alone. We talked about nothing while we waited for the doctors to come in and start the show. I didn't share with them all the possible side effects I had uncovered in my research. I was too embarrassed. I hoped they wouldn't find the Depends Adult Undergarments that I had stashed in the dresser that was partially blocking the 6 foot by 6 foot window. I was told that during the actual transplant, there's no way to tell how your body will react and uncontrolled bowel movements were fairly common. It's bad enough that you're fighting a horrible enemy who doesn't play by the rules. But to think of losing your basic dignity as a 32-year old adult and shitting your drawers in front of your mother was really taking this battle to a place it shouldn't ever be. This was going to be a street fight.

The Karmanos transplant ward is a separate, sterile area on the 10th floor of the Harper Hutzel hospital in downtown Detroit. It has a special air filtration system in each room to limit the potential for spreading germs or viruses. Without an immune system, this would be a medical necessity.

There was a sudden "whooooosh" as Dr. Payton, head of the transplant department, and his team came into my room. Apparently due to the special air filtration in the room the door had an airtight lock. I'm not a huge *Star Trek* fan, but I recall a similar sound when any of the doors on the ship opened or closed.

"Good morning, Don, are you ready to get this thing started?" I laughed my nerves away and said, "Why not. Seems I have a clear schedule this week anyway." He chuckled. I introduced my family. He instructed his lead nurse to begin the chemo IV. Too late, no turning back. I watched the first drip as it entered the line above me and followed it visually until it entered into my forearm.

The chemo flowed through my IV for approximately three hours. It was a particularly nasty cocktail designed to kill every cancer cell all at once. A bit like swatting a mosquito with a front end loader. However, after the first day of treatment, I really didn't feel all that bad. I spent the afternoon talking with my family and watching TV while they ran out for food. I always seem to find myself showing an outward confidence through these things for their sake. I would assure them that everything would be just fine. I hated to see the fear in my mother's eyes. It was so easy to read. It said, 'I'm not supposed to outlive my children.' It's a very sad sight to know you're causing this heartache even though you can rationally explain away the responsibility. That voice on the tape would run through my head, 'You caused this to happen. You stress too much. You don't exercise enough. If you'd been a better husband, you'd still be married.'

Thankfully my nurse, Sheila, wooshed into the room and interrupted me berating myself mentally. "OK, Don, I need you to get out of bed now. We're going for a walk," she said with a big grin. As I shuffled towards the door, rolling my IV pole along with me, she continued, "Every day I want you do four laps around the ward. You have to try and make sure you do at least four laps a day, OK?" I guesstimated the linear distance of the circular ward to be no more than 100 yards from start to finish. "Um, are you serious? That's not much of a feat. It's only going to take me like three minutes, or less." Sheila obliged my intended optimism with another warm smile. "So it's a deal then?" she asked. I shook her outstretched hand.

Later that evening, after I had sent my family to their hotels for the night, I settled in to watch some TV. I had never stayed overnight in a hospital before. Lucky me. But now I would have a 10-day sojourn here. I shut off the TV and began to drift off to sleep. *So far, this isn't that bad. I'll be all right.*

.......(whoooooosh!) A nurse I've never met comes waltzing into my room, robotically flipping on the light switch with her right hand on the way by. I looked at my clock. 12:07 a.m. As a general rule, I'm not a very good sleeper. That said, if I am sleeping and someone wakes me up, there'd better be a damn good reason. "What the hell is going on?" I barked at her.

I still wasn't fully alert.

"I need to take your vitals."

"Now? They took them this evening!"

"Your schedule calls for it every four hours."

"That's the dumbest thing I've ever heard!"

I was really pissed. Nobody told me about this 'schedule.' It takes me an hour to fall asleep on a good day. That means the next nine nights are going to be filled with, at best, three-hour naps, interrupted like clockwork by another nurse. It's true what they say, if you're sick, don't come to the hospital for rest.

After she had left my room, I had begun to think rationally again. *Of course they have to regularly check on patients. This is a transplant clinic. People die here. The nurses and doctors probably want to keep that to a minimum."* I felt badly about the attitude I gave her. I would learn to take the uninvited visits in stride from that night forward.

The next five days would repeat themselves like the movie *Groundhog's Day*. The doctor on staff would come into the room each morning around nine. He would ask me the same questions I had answered four hours ago. He would listen to my breathing with his stethoscope. Feel my pulse in my forearm for five seconds and then impart his wisdom, "You're doing great. Let's get you going on another round of treatment and we'll check in on you later today."

I would have three hours of chemo followed by 9-10 hours of watching crap TV or reading a book. I would purposely wait until Sheila's shift began before taking my laps around the ward. Day one was a breeze. I did maybe 20 laps before I simply got bored and stopped. I surmised that I had made my point to Sheila. *Four laps a day…HA!* But by day four or five, I would find myself struggling to complete a modest 10 laps. And on day six I tottered back into my room after only the 4th lap. I felt like a NASCAR driver rolling into "the pits" after careening off a wall and spinning through the infield. The chemo was taking its toll on my body. Breathing became labored due to a build-up of fluid in my lungs. My body was swelled to two times its normal size. The steroids they were giving me to keep me from puking all day were causing me to retain water. My face was huge. In addition, my skin had turned grey from anemia. And because my immune system was completely wiped out, there was nothing to fight the normal bacteria we all have on our skin. I had zits covering my entire face and body. I looked bad. I felt bad.

As bad as I looked, my family was a huge support. They never let on what a wreck I looked like on the outside. In fact I would have dismissed the impact of my appearance entirely, except for one particular visitor's reaction. On day five, quite unexpectedly, Sara walked into my room. We were not yet divorced and the sight of her caused my budding independence to quiver.

"How are you doing?" she asked as she cautiously advanced into the room.

"I'm doing all right. It's better than a sharp stick in the eye."

"You look good." She was a horrible liar. At that very moment I saw it in her eyes. She had come to see if she could handle getting back together with me as sick as I was. She was checking to see if she had the strength that would be needed. But her eyes had always been straight with me. She had no capacity to see me this sick. Her mind could not endure if she stayed by my side and had to watch me die. She was horribly afraid of my disease and what it was doing to me. I finally understood why we were no longer together. I finally made my peace with it.

At that moment a scene from the movie *Memphis Belle* played in my head. The movie's about World War II and specifically the crew aboard a bomber named the Memphis Belle. They had just flown through hours of enemy fire, watching many of their comrades' planes get shot down, leaving a trail of smoke to the ground. After dutifully dropping their bombs on the intended target, the captain made a comment to his crew along these lines: "Well boys, our job for the government is done. It's time to go home. Now we're flying for ourselves." That is exactly how I felt that moment back in the transplant ward. I was done fighting this battle for other people. I was done pretending things were fine so that friends, family and co-workers would worry less. This was my war. I alone would see myself through it to land safely back on my turf.

Finally with the 5 consecutive days of chemo behind me, I was now scheduled for two days of "rest." Here's how Dictionary.com describes the term rest:

rest1 - [rest]

—noun

1. the refreshing quiet or repose of sleep: *a good night's rest.*

2. relief or freedom, esp. from anything that wearies, troubles, or disturbs.

3. a period or interval of inactivity, repose, solitude, or tranquility: *to go away for a rest.*

I'm not sure who names the individual components of a stem cell transplant, but I think he/she must have bumped their head before they named this part "rest." They should have called it, "The part where we stop giving you chemo so that your body can revolt against what we've been doing to it. If you're not dead yet, we'll continue with the transplant." To me, there's little "solitude" or "tranquility" in a hospital bathroom puking your guts out while you wait for the next bout of diarrhea to present itself. But I digress...

The final segment of the transplant would immediately follow the two days of rest. Early on the morning of the 8th day, a female physician came whooshing into the room with a team of folks. There had to be at least five of them. The last two into the room were wheeling monitoring equipment and a defibrillator.

"We having a party, doc? Cause I can already tell I don't like the band," I said.

"Sort of, it's time for the last part, your transplant."

"Right on."

"I won't take time to introduce the team, but they're here because the frozen stem cells we're about to inject back into your body are so cold, we have to protect against cardiac arrest. Your body can react just like you've falling through a frozen lake."

"Seriously? They left that part out of the brochure."

I sat up in the bed to ready myself. My family stayed in the room. The thought of me dying right there in front of them didn't seem to be a deterrent. I was glad. I needed their support. I figured it was as a choice they had already made.

The doctor lifted a very large syringe, more like a turkey baster, filled with a slushy, yellowish cocktail of my frozen stem cells and a preserving agent. "Funny doc, that doesn't look like a margarita."

"Doesn't taste like one either. Oh, that reminds me, they mentioned the odor with this right?"

"Yes, can't wait."

It seems that the preserving agent they use to keep the stem cells alive while frozen, has an odor that oozes out of your pores after the transplant for several days. I had read that it smells like fish oil, not a particularly pleasant odor to me.

The doctor connected the turkey baster to my bendy straw and began pushing the frozen stem cells into me. At this point, I had come to the end of what I could handle emotionally. Maybe my family could stand to watch what was going to happen to me, but I couldn't. Often referred to as a "happy place", I mentally removed myself from what was happening to me.

In my mind I was now in Northern Michigan, at the Sleeping Bear National Dunes Park. On the western side of the National Park, the land plummets approximately 450 vertical feet to meet with Lake Michigan. With a length of 307 miles and a width of 118 miles, Lake Michigan seems more like an ocean to me. Due to the curvature of the Earth, you can't see the opposite shore, even from 450 feet up.

The winds blow across the lake from West to East. And these winds can be significant at times. As the waves roll in, they bring sand along with them and deposit it on the large beach that runs along the shores of Michigan. The constant wind then drives this sand onto land. Over perhaps thousands of years, one grain of sand at a time, the Sleeping Bear Dunes have been formed.

Imagine a hill, so steep that when you run down it, you're virtually weightless. But there's no grass on this hill, no trees. Only sand and rocks. You run to the bottom, jumping and spanning distances of 20-30 feet with each leap. You spin in the air and laugh like a child. It's been decades since you've felt like this. Even with this superhuman leaping ability, it still takes you nearly five minutes to get to the bottom.

Now you are rewarded with the chance to catch your breath and play in the icy waters of Lake Michigan. You soak your feet, cooling them from the friction of your descent, until they go numb and you have to get out. You grab a stone, worn perfectly smooth and flat by the waves. You attempt to skip it across the water. It only skips twice because you've never really been very good at that. You tire of playing and decide you'd like to head back up to the car now.

You look up the hill, leaning backwards and bending your neck as far back as it will go to allow a view of the top. You notice a reddish line that seems to run across the very middle of the hill. You think it's something put there for the tourists. Actually it's a natural layer of clay, set down thousands of years before by Mother Nature. It's just weird to see it exactly half way up the hill.

You begin your ascent. The first two minutes you're climbing, upright and still happy. But within the first 50 feet, the hill becomes so steep you have to bend over on all fours or you will fall over backwards. Adding to the difficulty, the sand beneath you slides down the hill and you lose half of every step back to the hill.

Undaunted, you continue to climb, stopping every 10-20 feet amazed that you're breathing as heavy as you are. Your leg muscles are so swelled with blood it's hard to move them. You wait for a few minutes, resting as if you just sprinted a mile. At some point, pride will make you continue the climb. You repeat this process 10 or 15 more times. You're feeling dizzy and lightheaded. You have to rest. *What the hell am I doing here*, you ask yourself. It's the beginning of a conversation you'll have for the rest of the 40-minute climb. It will become an increasingly desperate conversation.

After resting for a minute, still gasping for air, you lift your head expecting to see the top of the hill. But instead, about 75 feet above, you see a wide red line running across your path. "Oh shit!" you say out loud. *I'm not even halfway there yet!* Fear begins to interrupt your vacation for the first time. *I can't get to the car if I don't go up. It's like a 5-mile walk if I go back down and have to go along the beach. And then I'd have to call for someone to come pick me up.*

You decide to continue, determined to get to that red line. 10 more feet climbed and you rest. This time for only 30 seconds before you start again. 15 more feet and another rest. Climb. Rest. Climb. Rest. You cross the red line and collapse. But sitting is difficult because of the steepness of the hill. Even though you're sitting down, facing Lake Michigan, you have to dig yourself in and really hold on to the hill. The sand shifts underneath you.

You begin to review your life to this point. The decisions you've made along the way. People you've met and some you no longer see. *I really should call my old high school buddy more often. It's been two years since we've spoken and I still haven't been to North Carolina to visit him yet.*

You swear off smoking. You contemplate your relationship with God. You worry about retirement. This dune climb produces raw emotion. And it is very overwhelming.

At some point the reality sets in that you're only halfway done, so you begin your climb again. 10-15 feet at a time, and then rest. The cycle seems never-ending. You're now about ¾ of the way up the hill and you notice two things. First, the steepness of the hill has actually increased! The last 25% of the climb is going to be the hardest, but strangely you know you'll make it.

And second, you look over to your left and you see me. I'm in a seated position facing the lake, muscles tensing to keep from sliding. You've found me in my "happy place." I have a huge smile on my face. As I look over the water, all I can see is blue. The sky is blue and the water is blue. Some 200 feet below, a seagull coasts at its normal altitude. It seems more like a white fly from this height. The wind is steady, but the breeze helps whisk away the sweat of the ascent. The sun warms you from the inside out. It's deafeningly quiet. "My life is perfect," I say under my breath. "No matter what happens with my cancer, I have no regrets. It doesn't matter how long it takes to climb this, or any other hill. I'm a climber. I get it now." The meaning of life, as it applies to me, is clear. And that epiphany invokes a warming confidence that produces a mild high inside of me. This is my happy place.

As I clung to the face of the dune, taking it all in, the clean air is replaced by an overwhelming smell of creamed corn with a hint of fish oil. I hear a voice shout down from the top of the hill. "OK, this is the last syringe. We collected so many stem cells from you that this is an extra, but we might as well use it. Better safe than sorry." And with that, I was back in my hospital bed, watching the doctor push the slushy concoction into my chest. She was finished. It was over. I said nothing. I reached for the shallow basin they had set beside me, sat up and vomited like never before. I had no control over the eruption and it seemed to start from a place inside of me quite unfamiliar. But I was one and done. I wiped my mouth clean. The doctor was extremely calm and supportive. "That's OK, Hun. That's perfectly normal and we expect it. Actually, you did amazingly well. Better than anyone I've ever seen!" In some weird way, I took pride in that fact. It's amazing how people can be affected by simple compliments. Later that day I was discharged from the hospital... sort of.

CHAPTER 10
Transplant Recovery

Two weeks prior, I was explaining the transplant process to Cousin Dave. "Following this transplant, my body's immune system will be completely wiped out. I'll have no natural defenses against germs or viruses." So when they let me out, I have to stay at these medical apartments, right next to the hospital, for like two weeks.

"How come," Cousin Dave asked. He's the kind of person who listens intently, with only a very few questions as he gathers info.

"So I'm always close to the Emergency Room if I need it and because I have to report into the lab every morning at seven for blood work."

I had something else I needed to explain to Dave. Rather, something I needed to ask him. I was dreading my own question and his possible response to it. The hospital requires that you have a full-time caregiver with you 24 hours a day for this 2-week period. That person is there to make sure you get up and get to your appointments. They watch you for serious signs of illness. And finally, they are there to be your liaison to the outside world, because you are now a complete shut-in until your immune system regrows. I found this last requirement to be the most awkward of all of them. I wasn't comfortable asking my parents to do it. They were having their own health concerns. Not to mention they're from a tiny town in Northern Michigan called Petoskey, some 300 miles north of here. They don't like big cities, especially Detroit. So now who do I turn to?

Being recently divorced, this situation made me feel alone. I saw for the first time that my life was filled with fair-weather friends, the kind who diligently managed their own agendas and couldn't be counted on for this critical assignment. As I thought through the short list of names of people I could even ask to do this, I realized there was really only one person...Cousin Dave. He and I had always been very close. Part cousins, part brothers, part best friends.

I hated that I had to ask him this. It's a huge responsibility to have to take another person's life in your hands and be their protector.

I figured I'd just float it by him nonchalantly and if he didn't pick it up and run with it, I'd just tell the doctors I didn't have anyone. Most likely they would have cancelled my transplant though. "Dave, I need to run something by you." Apparently he could tell from my tone that it was something fairly serious. He stopped cleaning out the monstrous cage in the living room that housed his pet iguana, Daedalus. No doubt, Dave was a bachelor, thru and thru.

"What's that?" he asked, sticking to his two-word line of questioning.

"Well…I have to have a caregiver after the transplant for two weeks, non-stop. I'm gonna need someone to take care of me cause I won't be able to do it on my own."

"I'll do it," he said almost cutting me off.

"I think you might need to know a little more about what I need you to do before you agree to it."

"Doesn't matter. Whatever you need, I got ya covered."

I was completely overcome with emotions. What an amazingly selfless act I had just witnessed! "Dave, you rock! I really appreciate it."

"No problem, Bro," and he went back to cleaning the cage.

"Oh, one more thing…I want you and Kevin to shave my head."

"What," he clamored. "Why would we do that?"

"I'm gonna lose it all anyway and I'd rather take control."

Just then my cousin Kevin came strolling in from work.

"Hey Kevin, I want you and Dave to shave my head tonight."

"Right on," he said without missing a beat. "Let me grab a beer and the scissors."

What they didn't know was that I was terrified to have my head shaved. My earliest childhood memories were of friends, family members and classmates teasing me about how big my ears were. I used to grow my hair long to try and cover them up and I would use the muscles on the side of my head to try and hold them back whenever anyone else was around. I had unconsciously carried this fear of judgment all the way through my life and up to the minute that Kevin turned on those clippers. This was more than a natural fear of losing one's hair; I was staring down a weight that I had carried for far too long. For the record, my cousin Kevin has zero chance of ever becoming a barber! ;)

Thrombocytopenia was going to be the first major risk I faced after being discharged to the medical apartments. This is a serious condition that refers to extremely low platelet counts in the blood; brought on by the mega-doses of chemo I had received. It's the official term when someone says you've lost your immune system. And there are a huge amount of precautions you have to take and things you have to avoid. Your body can no longer protect itself against simple germs or viruses that a normal, healthy person would be bombarded with daily. Whenever I was around people, I had to wear a surgical mask covering my nose and mouth. This would hopefully protect me from any airborne viruses or bacteria. I wasn't allowed in public places, like grocery stores, movie theatres or restaurants. I was forbidden to pump my own gas into my car. This was to keep the toxins in the gasoline vapors out of my sensitive lung tissue. I was not allowed to eat fresh fruits or vegetables, since they often carry germs and bacteria. And finally, I couldn't use pepper on anything I ate since pepper naturally contains a boatload of bacteria and fungi that could lead to major complications for someone in my condition.

Armed with my marching orders and a standing appointment at the lab every morning at seven o'clock, Dave and I moved into the medical apartment in downtown Detroit. We walked in the door and I was shocked at the conditions! It was run down and dirty beyond belief. The carpeting was stained with I don't-wanna-know-what. The walls in the kitchen were covered in black marks, like the kind a black-soled shoe would leave on a wooden floor if you intentionally tried to scuff it. The light fixture in the center of the kitchen was filthy and there were dozens of dead flies in its bowl, completely visible when the light was on. The handles of the refrigerator were broken off and sitting on top of it. The paint on the walls of the bathroom was chipping off. I was willing to put money on the fact that it was still lead-based paint. "Dave, this place is an absolute shithole!"

"I know. You should have seen it before I cleaned it."

"What?!?"

"Yeah, I found out a couple hours before your release which one was yours and got the keys. I wanted to make sure you were all set up and comfortable. It was so nasty, I ran to a party store, bought cleaning supplies and scrubbed the place down."

"Damn," I said and shook my head. I was moved by his help and caring and at the same time disgusted by the condition of this "medical apartment." *This is nothing but an insurance reimbursed flophouse,* I thought to myself. Based on all the thought and work Dave had done, I decided to stay and try to make the best of it. It turned out to be just one night.

The next morning we got up, I prepared to go to the lab all day, and Dave got ready for work. You see, he worked at Chrysler at their world headquarters, some 40 miles north of the hospital. But his house was only about 10 miles from where he worked. So not only was he handling all the caretaking responsibilities for me, he had to drive an extra 60 miles a day while doing it. When he finally was set to head out the door, I said, "Dave, we're not staying here again...ever. I'm going home to stay in my own bed. My apartment is infinitely cleaner and healthier than this place!"

"I agree with you there. But how will you get your doctors to OK it?"

"I'll take care of it. I'll give you a call when I'm cut loose for the day and whenever you can come back and pick me up will be great."

"Sounds good but I'll be staying on your couch to keep an eye on you."

"It's a deal."

I arrived at the blood lab at 7:30 a.m., not really knowing what to expect. I was met with forms to fill out, waiting rooms to sit in, and bureaucracy to deal with. Around 9:45 they finally called my name and led me back behind the mystery door. In the treatment area, there were about a dozen or so "one-up cubicles" as I coined them. Each cube had a hospital bed, a 50-year old, square, wooden chair with red vinyl upholstery, and a 12 inch TV that is mounted to a steel arm which swings over the bed so you can see it while lying down.

By 10 a.m. the nurse on staff had drawn my blood and sent it for analysis to another lab in the basement of the hospital. Once they identified which normal elements I was low on, they would pipe the needed essentials into my IV and then send me home. Mostly it was things like potassium, or magnesium, A-blood, or A-platelets. Sounds quick, right? Well my results finally came back from the basement lab at 12:30. It would be another two hours after that before I was released on this first day. But at least it was over, and I would sleep in my own bed tonight. One visit down, nine to go. *Maybe less,* I thought. *I'm way healthier than their average patient. I bet I can wrap this up in six total visits.*

So that night, Dave and I sat around my apartment, watched TV and shot the shit. We grilled some steaks, no pepper on mine, and had a fun time. It was nice to have someone to talk about all of this to. Eventually, I got sleepy, so I went to bed and Dave crashed on the couch till the morning. When we got up the next morning, I let Dave off the hook. Mostly I was relieving myself of the guilt that my illness was having such a negative impact on his life. "Dave, there's really no reason why you have to stay here. Your house is only 10 minutes away. We both have cell phones. If I need something, I can call you. Why don't you just stay home and we'll put you on call?"

The look in Dave's eyes was unique. I imagined it was similar to a mountain skier who had been trapped by an avalanche, but could now hear digging above and see a ray of light breaking through the surface of the snow. His tentative look seemed to expose his shame of the fact that he liked this idea. It was more convenient for him, but in some way by agreeing to it, he would be letting me down and going back on the promise he had made. I was really going to have to sell this idea hard.

"Seriously though, Dave, I'm not new to this cancer thing. I can handle this. I'd feel better if I knew you were home comfortable and just checking in on me daily or something."

"Well, you'd have to call me every morning as soon as you woke up so I knew you were OK?"

"No problem."

"And I'd still come over every day after work to check on you myself."

"Fine."

"And I'll take your car to fill it with gas when it's low and take your grocery list to the store every couple of days. Then, if you need anything else, you'll just call when I'm on my way over?"

"Sounds like a much smarter plan to me, brotha."

So for the next eight days, my routine was set. Each morning at 5:30 I would wake up to my alarm, a sound that I particularly loathe by the way. I would climb into the shower, barely awake. Once I was just about ready to leave for the hospital, I would call Dave and let him know everything was on track and running smoothly. Then I would drive approximately 45-50 minutes down to the hospital, depending on traffic. It happened to be January in Detroit, and a particularly frigid January at that. Each morning the temperature hovered around −10 F, with a wind-chill making it feel like −30 below. Half of my commute each morning was spent just thawing my body from being in a frozen car in these temperatures.

I would park in the parking structure next to the hospital, put on my hospital mask, and make the 3-minute walk over to the main building. After being delayed some 30-45 minutes in the waiting room each day, I was then brought back to an unoccupied "cubicle" in the lab's treatment area. I would watch daytime TV to help pass the time. They only got 5 channels in the hospital, and the lesser of all evils to me was TNT. I watched several year's worth of *E.R., Charmed* and *Law & Order* reruns over that time. To this day, I still know every note to the *Law & Order* theme song they play in the beginning. It's not something I'm proud of and I can't seem to bring myself to watch the show since.

The nurses would test my blood, fill me up on whatever I was low on and send me home. I would try to take a nap and do some meditation while I waited for Dave to come over after work. If I needed gas in my car, or food from the grocery store, he'd take care of it when he got there. Then we'd make some dinner and just chill watching sports or The Comedy Channel in the evening. This short time in the evening was my only mental respite and would allow me to pretend my life was normal. But the next morning would always come too soon.

On the tenth day my blood test showed that my stem cells had started to reform bone marrow. This process is known as engraftment. Basically, if it doesn't work, you have to live your life without an immune system. And it would be a short life after that. I was overjoyed to hear the news. I was filled with energy and decided right then and there that I had won this battle and kicked this cancer's tail once-and-for-all. And to prove it, I would live my remaining life with a gusto never before seen. At least not by me.

CHAPTER 11
"Fuck You, I'm Still Alive!"

After a few months of hanging around in my one bedroom apartment by myself, my test results showed that I was as healthy as an average 19-year old. My immune system had grown back to full strength. But out of nowhere, something else had grown as well. A huge chip on my shoulder. At first it started as a zest to live life to its fullest, a seemingly innocent and noble lifestyle. But gradually it turned darker. Fueled by drugs and alcohol, I was about to set a world-record partying pace. I didn't care who got caught up in my wake. It was a period in my life that I came to refer to as "Fuck you! I'm still alive!"

Remission has a funny way of affecting some people. Even more so, a second remission. And I'm certainly no exception. I had been battling on and off with my cancer for about two years now. I'd also been battling, mostly on, with my thoughts and emotions. In retrospect, the emotional toll that I was under was like a black mold hiding inside of a house's walls. You can scrub those walls with bleach all you want. But if you don't change the conditions that are causing the mold to grow in the first place, you better be comfortable with seeing little black spots all over your new wallpaper.

During my second remission, I started out with my head held high; appreciating every minute of time I was given. I gave thanks for every new day and looked forward to the people and experiences that I would encounter. As far as my physical appearance went, surprisingly, I received so many compliments from women of all sorts. They all wanted the same thing....to touch my bald head. Literally, at least twice a day, a woman I didn't know would ask to touch my head. I loved it. It reminded me of all the teasing I endured throughout my youth. It was a release from all the nasty comments I had heard and dragged with me for my entire adult life. The more attention they gave, the more I wanted.

I further defined my new mantra, "Now is the time!" I decided that if I was ever going to do anything, it had to be done now, not later. Now, I'm not talking about bull riding, or jumping out of an airplane, but I made sure if something interested me, I tried it. I got back into downhill skiing for the first time in about 10 years. The following summer, I started playing beach volleyball several times per week. I bought a hunting rifle and a shotgun and got back out into the great outdoors in Northern Michigan. I bought a new fishing pole for the same reason. I was getting back to my roots and trying to live, as Dr. Phil would say, as my authentic self. And I felt incredible. I was sleeping soundly every night, something I hadn't done since I was a teenager. I was thankful for everything in my life and was an extremely happy person. I convinced my company to let me come back to work early. I had been on long-term disability and I felt guilty for sitting around at home and getting paid damn near as much as I did when I worked.

Soon, I started going out at night with my friends, at the time, to make new social connections. I had always wanted a "go-fast car" so I bought a Corvette. It was black-on-black with a removable glass top. For you Vette fans, it was a 2000, C6 version. I had upgraded it with chrome wheels and chrome accents on most of the outside of the car. And to complete my ride, a personalized licensed plate for the back, "MOVEOVA." Incredibly cheesy, I understand. But it fit the way I was living my life at the time. No one was gonna stop my roll. Frankly, I just didn't give a shit. I rationalized that my behavior was just my desire to have fun and live life carefree. But over time it showed its true self: gluttony, irresponsibility, and plain disregard of the future.

In hindsight, I believe that my problem centered on the fact that I didn't love the person I was. I was too worried about what other people thought about me and was concerned with impressing them. But then, I had always been that way. Did I buy the car for me, or to impress others? Did I valet the car at every bar and pay an extra $20 each time to have it parked up front because I was too impatient to wait for it to arrive at the end of the night? I was starting to live to be the life of the party. I had such an external appearance of self-confidence that I could attract just about anyone into my world. But inside, I was moving farther and farther away from my authentic self. I was horribly lonely after all that I had been through. I was a black hole, and beware those that got close.

I know now that being a cancer survivor takes a huge emotional toll on you in many ways. "Fuck you, I'm still alive!" was a direct result of one of those ways.

During the treatment process, I grew to hate being the center of attention. Every doctor's visit, every treatment session, every CT scan, every PET scan, every cardiac test, every pulmonary function test, every conversation with an old friend you haven't seen since treatment started, every family reunion, every foursome of golf, every small or large get-together. All of the people in your life want to know how you are doing. They mean well and only want the best for you, but they <u>need</u> some validation from you about your current status.

I still get one question more than any other, even up to the day of this writing, "How's your health?" This simple little, well-intended, 3-word question has become my personal nemesis. It forces you to reflect on your cancer, no matter how much you've tried to move past it. It keeps you tied to your illness. With a fragile emotional state, it's all that's required to send you off onto an internal roll coaster ride that's called "I wonder when it's coming back." In addition, it seemed to keep me tied to hopelessness. I didn't care about the future, I guess because deep down I didn't really think I had one anyways. Cancer became an emotional trap for me. I fell into the "victim's role" all too easily. I used cancer as an excuse, internally and externally. It was a reason to do whatever I wanted, whenever I wanted. It was a reason not to do anything I didn't want. It was a reason not to try. It was a catchall.

And so I spent the summer after my transplant living a short-term life. I partied perhaps five days per week on average. My social circle had to ebb and flow, temporarily replacing members when they were unavailable or unable to keep the pace. We golfed during the day, even during the workweek. We would usually have 6-8 beers each during the four hours it took us to golf. We would finish around 6 p.m. and usually head out to dinner somewhere close as a group. All-you-could-eat crab legs specials were a favorite. After dinner, we would adjourn to our separate homes, to shower and relax for a bit. About 9 p.m. we would regroup at one of dozens of bars in Royal Oak. For those who haven't been there, Royal Oak, Michigan, is like a mini Daytona Beach. There are dozens of bars/clubs and even more restaurants all within walking distance.

So we would drink at one of these fine establishments from 9 p.m.-2 a.m. (legal cutoff for serving alcohol in Michigan). Most nights, we would consume perhaps another 10-15 beers each in this time.

Following "last call" the streets would now be full of intoxicated drivers, doing their best to avoid the militant patrols of the Royal Oak Police Department.

Now, depending on what night of the week it was, would dictate what happened from here for some of us. If it were a Thursday, Friday or Saturday, a much smaller group of us would head to an after-hours club. This was a quasi-secret spot, with a private members list, where the ultra hard partiers go to dance to techno/rave music until 4 a.m. It's a spot where straight folks like us partied in close quarters to the often unseen gay crowd of Detroit, and the seemingly gangster crowd as well. This was not an extremely safe place to be, and we knew it.

The only after-hours club was in the city of Detroit, on 6 Mile Road. It was called Numbers. Shootings were not that uncommon around this place. You could actually feel when tensions started running high in the club. The DJ would stop the music and the owner would shut the place down early and lock the doors. Not the place for three white boys from the suburbs to be after dark in retrospect.

Because it's past 2 a.m., these transient locations can not sell alcohol. At the bar in the front of the building, all they sell is water or Red Bull. But it's on the dance floor or around the pool tables where the real products are moved. Cocaine, weed, Ecstasy, you name it. We were there for the coke. The more often we came and the more we got to know the dealers, the better the quality we got. We would buy a small bag of it, perhaps a tablespoon's worth, for $60. And that would usually last the three of us a week.

Cocaine is an interesting drug. I tell people that if you've never tried it, DON'T! It's not like it has some overwhelming buzz that puts you in the captain's seat of a rocket ship or anything like that. It makes you alert, awake, and absolutely happy with your life. It's a very false happiness, but who cares? That's why it was such a perfect escape for me at the time. Emotionally, I could not handle my life anymore and coke was a way out, if only for a few hours each time.

Another effect of coke is overt alertness. But for me, that effect was the same as insomnia. I've always been a lousy sleeper to start with. But this stuff wouldn't leave me alone. We'd be doing coke at the bar, and by the time I got home, around 6 a.m., I was still wide awake. Often it would take me until 10 a.m. just to fall asleep. I nailed sleeping bags over my apartment blinds so that the room would stay pitch black to help me sleep. Usually I would only sleep for a couple of hours and then the guilt of blowing off another workday would cause me to get up.

You see, I was an 8a.m.- 6p.m. professional sales rep in the Information Technology field. But I use the term "professional" very loosely to describe this period of my life. My partying caused me to skip meetings and fall behind in my duties. My sales had hit an all-time low during this period, but I really didn't care. Not only was I burning the candle at both ends, I had a blowtorch to the middle of the sucker.

CHAPTER 12
Relapse #2

My party life continued until one day in the early Fall. I had gone to get my usual CT scans done, three months after my last tests showed all clear. I was in one of Dr. Jeff's exam rooms, waiting for him to come in and give me the results. He opened the door and walked slowly into the room. Now mind you, he usually flung the door open and slid right into the room. He didn't sit down on his stool by the counter where he always sat. Rather, he stood only a step or two in front of me. He reviewed the chart one more time, as if to hope he had read it incorrectly the first six times. He lowered the chart in front of him and said, "Your tests are positive for cancer again. And it's spread to your lungs as well as your liver. You also have a very large mass that has returned to your chest." With that, he stepped over to me, helped me stand up, and hugged me, as if to say, "I'm sorry I couldn't save you." I froze emotionless.

Seeing that kind of concern from him floored me. Inside, I was like a spinning plate that had slowed on its pole too much and had begun to wobble. I just sat there…not sure how long…pondering his words and approach. *This man, whom I completely respect and trust, just gave me the kiss of death and has written me off. I must be in serious trouble here!* I decided I had to try to pull myself together.

"What are my options now?"

"Well, you can do the allogeneic stem cell transplant where we use your Brother Mike's cells since he's a perfect match. That's what I would recommend at this point. Or we can resume chemo treatment with the intent to keep you alive as long as possible."

I know from previous research that using someone else's cells is much riskier. The safest bet is with a significantly positive HLA match, and that usually means a sibling or twin. Even if I did use cells that are a good match, there's still somewhere around a 30% chance that I could die from the transplant in the first

100 days. It seems that the donor cell's natural defenses could see my body as an enemy and attack it. This is called graft versus host disease and it's serious business.

Even if the transplant's complications didn't lead to my death, the list of possible side effects was dumbfounding. Lung disease, kidney disease, infection, liver disease, heart disease, secondary cancers, cataracts, inflammation of the mouth and intestinal linings, skin rashes, hardening of the skin, jaundice, and diarrhea. This may happen all at once and then slowly resolve, called acute GVHD. Or it may roll out slowly, happening over years, and never going away, called chronic GVHD. I really had a hard time accepting that a life of dealing with these kinds of chronic problems could be better than where I was right now. After all, I felt incredible, except for this stinking cough. *No, I'm not doing this yet. That's a Hail Mary pass as far as I'm concerned, and I still have half of a playbook left.*

"Here's what I want to do," I said. "We're gonna start chemo again, this time our intent is to go slow and low, not having any particular end in sight. I want you to go into your tool box of chemo, and pull out the smallest hammer that has a positive effect." Chemo, in my opinion, has always been about using the biggest hammer, as fast as possible, without killing the patient. But for me, at this point, I just wanted to use it as a regular maintenance drug, and keep the cancer from spreading. I was much more interested in quality of life now, not longevity. Dr. Jeff was nodding and smiling now. He was back on board.

"Right, and we could treat the big spot on your chest with radiation too since we've never used that on you before."

"Ok, now we're talking," I said.

CHAPTER 13
Treatment, Round #3

This is the point in time, I think, where a lot of people go down hill quickly. They *"lose their battle with cancer."* But I think it's because they lose their <u>hope</u>. I'm not telling you that I stared this climb in the face and thought, "piece of cake." Not even close. In fact, this whole journey I'd spoken confidently, while inside my every thought was of being terrified to die from this. But in my heart, I knew that only I could cure myself. I had the power inside of me. But I just didn't fully understand how to put that power to use quite yet. It's like knowing all the words to a song. It doesn't mean you can karaoke. It takes practice to become meaningful.

So here I was, about to start my third round of treatment in as many years. A few months prior to this, I had met a beautiful woman, named Tina, at a bar in downtown Detroit and we had been dating very seriously. She was a nurse and could charm the coldest heart with her smile and childlike laugh. She had long, natural blond hair and stood no taller than 5' 3". I wasn't really looking for a girlfriend when we met, but that is exactly what I ended up getting. And although this would turn out to be the most unhealthy relationship I would ever have, it was one of the most inspiring times of my life.

Tina and I spent increasingly large amounts of time together. Undetectably, she was pulling me away from my friends and the life I was living. I went from being at the bar to all hours of the night five times per week, down to having dinner/drinks and home by 10 p.m. twice a week. And I couldn't have been happier. In fact, it was her that helped me explore new areas of fitness, spirituality/religion and family life. But I dare not paint too rosy of a picture for this relationship. Not by a looooooong shot.

Tina was conniving, controlling, belittling, emotionally abusive, and holier-than-thou. At times, she would give me just enough positive emotion and affection to keep me close. I didn't realize it at the time, but I had begun to make excuses to explain her behavior. Really what I was doing was rationalizing why I stayed with her. I couldn't see it, but she had taken control of me. My friends saw it though. To this day, they still refer to her as "The Cult." She was controlling me like a cult leader would.

It seems that I was stuck in an emotional tug of war, and no matter who would win, I was going to lose. On one side, I had a tumultuous relationship that I was struggling to keep afloat. If I was successful, I could expect a lifetime of sadness, sorrow, arguments and suspicion. If I lost, my emotions would have sunk even lower, further weakening me against the ever-advancing cancer in my body.

At first, Tina was very supportive, at least to my face. I held the cancer at bay, even made up some ground on it. But eventually, Tina's true feelings made it to the surface. She never had any intention of standing by me. A small part of me thinks she was using me for money and support through a "rough" time in her life.

We argued more often each week. One evening she started in on me by saying, "It's not fair to me that my future is uncertain and difficult because of your illness. No woman should have to settle for that." The conversation escalated until eventually she stormed out of my apartment, the one I was letting her and her three siblings stay in rent-free. She turned and screamed at me, "I hope you DO die!!!" and slammed the door on her way out.

Ok, I know what you're thinking. This chick just shit on you! I can't think of something much colder than that to say to someone. I'm not going to say that I immediately broke it off, because I didn't. I wish I had. In fact, this insipid relationship smoldered for months after.

Eventually, I reached my emotional breaking point. And man, am I glad I finally did. I dumped her for good. I was a wreck for months after, but I survived.

This terrible relationship would help me learn that I wasn't putting myself first in my own mind. If I didn't respect and love myself first, how the hell can I ask another person to do it? And if I loved myself, I sure as hell wouldn't have dated her more than once. After all, I am the only person responsible for my happiness. This relationship had actually proved to be a turning point for me, an epiphany if you will. For that I owe Tina a "thank you." It's possible that my emotional growth from that train wreck is what eventually saved my life. Or at least that's how I choose to remember it. There must have been some reason for my time with her.

Although I was stronger post-Tina, I still wasn't where I needed to be. I wanted to be the picture of happiness. I worked out every day. I ate the right things. I smiled and laughed a lot. But inside, I was a wreck of emotions.

In his book *Beating Cancer with Nutrition*, Dr. Patrick Quillin states, "What you're eating is not as important as what's eating you." Now I think that speaks volumes if you stop and think about it. Here's a nutritionist, with a Ph.D. no less, who wrote a book about curing your cancer with the right nutrition. He then comes out and essentially says, 'eating healthy ain't gonna fix the damage your negative thoughts are doing my friend. You'd better get your mind straight first.'

But I couldn't seem to control my negative thoughts anymore. The more I worried about my cancer, the more anxiety I felt. Eventually, I would get anxiety over my anxiety because I knew that it was weakening my immune system. I pictured the cancer advancing, unfettered by my body's natural defenses. I would sweat profusely while having my anxious thoughts. All of this stress would cause my skin to breakout, both on my face, as well as all over my back. Now I wasn't comfortable taking my shirt off in public anymore. In fact, I was disgusted at the thought. I had a constant tightness in my chest, frequently accompanied by a dark, heavy feeling of "butterflies." I would have a headache about once a day and I rapidly developed acid reflux. I really believed that I, myself, was responsible for my cancer. If my emotional stress and negative thoughts could produce all of these visible ailments on my outside, it must be doing the same to my insides. I knew that my thoughts were my own enemy, but I could not seem to change them with any lasting effect.

So I was on my own again, facing another round of chemo. This time they would add radiation to the mix to treat a huge mass of tumor in my chest. I actually don't believe that my doctors thought they could save me. I think they were just trying to buy me more time in their minds. Seeing that in their eyes and hearing it in their words was actually a blessing to me. If not for any other reason than spite, I was going to beat this thing again just to prove them wrong. After all, my whole cancer career has been about showing everyone that statistics don't apply to individuals.

I went into my chemo treatments with a playful attitude. One of the chemo drugs that I received, Gemcitabine, is known to cause sclerosis, or hardening of the veins that it goes into. My nurse said, "You don't have any good veins left on the tops of your arms. I'm going to have to use the ones on the bottoms of your forearms."

"Nope, can't let you do that, Teresa. Sand volleyball league starts next week and I need that part of my arm to bump the ball. You'll have to make the others work, or check out my feet."

She was a bit taken aback by me placing more importance on volleyball than on my life-saving treatments. But to me, volleyball, and more accurately, the **good** times left in my life, were more therapeutic than any drug cocktail she could drip into my IV. After all, this wasn't my first rodeo with chemo. I'd already had these medications and they didn't stop the disease before. I'm not positive that I was expecting much more from them this time around. I stuck to my belief that it was my internal attitude that was the X-factor here and ultimately what was going to save or sink me. I made sure that I was having fun with everything I did. If it wasn't fun, I didn't do it.

While waiting in the exam room one chemo day, I decided I would start messing with the residents who invariably would come in to take a whole history on me. This was a teaching hospital and these "work ups" were for their training, not my treatment. I could have gotten irritated by them and just insisted that only Dr. Jeff would be allowed to work with me. But where's the fun in that? I decided I was going to start having some entertainment at their expense, but wasn't sure how I would do it.

The day before my radiation was set to begin, I was sitting on the exam table in Dr. Jeff's office. There's a knock at the door. A young Middle Eastern woman in a short white lab coat walks in. I knew she was a resident cause you can tell their rank by the length of their lab coats. Residents get the shortest ones, barely coming down to their waist. Doctors always get the longest, hanging below the knee.

Showtime! I thought.

"Hi Mr. Wilheeb, I'm Dr. Harkenflarfer. Dr. Margolis will be in shortly, but I need to examine you first."

"OK, go ahead."

"Now it says here in your chart that you have Stage IV Hodgkin's Lymphoma."

"What?!? What the hell is that?!!"

Stunned, she paused, took a step backwards and then said, "…well, it's cancer."

"OH MY GOD!!! ARE YOU TELLING ME I HAVE HAD CANCER ALL THIS TIME AND I'M JUST NOW FINDING OUT ABOUT IT?!? AND WHAT THE HELL KIND OF WAY IS THAT TO BREAK THE NEWS TO SOMEONE?!? OH MY GOD!!.....<snicker to myself>…no, I'm just kidding around."

Her face goes from transparent white to a deep red in one second flat. *How's that for a teaching school,* I thought to myself. Expect the unexpected. Patients are crazy. I am entertained, albeit at her expense, but I don't care. I could rationalize this bit of mental playtime no matter how emotionally scarred I left these newbies.

CHAPTER 14
Radiation Therapy

Bright and early the next morning, I found myself in the radiation department of Beaumont Hospital. It is in the lower level of the building, but surprisingly well lit and cheery in atmosphere. There were interesting works of art on the walls and a huge fish tank teaming with exotic fish in the lobby.

Today would be my consult visit where they would explain how all of this worked. I met with Dr. Over Booked first. I call him that because I would only see him twice, for three minutes each time, over the course of my treatments. Dr. Over Booked explained the process to me, in broad brush strokes. "The first thing we do today, Mr. Wilhelm, is make a mask of your face and neck. We use this mask to secure your head during the treatments to ensure the most accurate results. Your actual treatments will begin tomorrow morning."

"How does the treatment work," I asked.

"Well, it's just like an ex-ray machine, only instead of turning the machine on for a 1-2 second blast, we leave it on for a couple of minutes."

"Hmmm, me thinks thou doth leave out all the gory details, Doc."

He chuckles and loosens up a bit. "Well, of course there are side effects of the treatment as we'll discuss, but the time you spend in this office is a breeze. You'll see."

I was encouraged by his confidence and swagger. But I'd been oversold in these new situations before. *Remember the bone marrow biopsy test?* I thought. After all, I was a weathered veteran of this cancer gig and my respect had to be earned at this point.

Shortly afterwards one of the nurses' assistants came to get me and led me back for 'mask creation.' I'm telling you now, this was one of the strangest parts of my treatments to date. Not necessarily in a bad way, I just wonder who in the hell thought up this process in the first place.

See here's how it goes: The staff had me take my shirt off and lie down on the exam table. All of my stress had caused the skin on my back to break out, what I affectionately referred to as my "backne." But I digress. The nurse said to me, "We're going to take wet strips of a white material and lay them over your face and neck. After about 20 minutes, the strips will dry to something like plaster. Your job is to lie perfectly still without talking."

"Doesn't sound too bad. I think I can do that."

So I laid there on the table as the nurse and her assistant layered piece after wet piece of material over my face, careful to leave holes for my eyes and nostrils. It felt cold and gooey as they put it on. When they covered my nose and mouth, I had a weird sensation like I was being mummified. I was becoming a bit short of breath from the slight claustrophobic feeling of having my head encased. I started to sweat nervously.

After 20 minutes or so, the nurse lifted and pried the completely hardened mask off my face.

"Isn't it cool looking?" she said as she handed the mask to me."

"Yeah, a little bit," I said. "What are these two metal clips on the sides for?"

"That's what we use to secure the mask to the treatment table so your head and neck remain perfectly still."

"Ah, OK. This is all very strange to me still."

"Don't worry, after your first treatment tomorrow morning this will all make sense to you. Compared to what you've been through so far, I think you'll be pleasantly surprised at how easy this part is."

"You should be in sales cause you've actually got me looking forward to my first radiation treatment!" We all shared a laugh.

"OK, Donald," she said. "Now I need you to lay back on the table. We need to mark your chest with guidelines so we can make sure you're aligned exactly the same way for each treatment."

"OK, how do you do that? Do I not get to shower for the next three weeks or what?"

She smiled and said, "No. Have you ever had a tattoo?"

"Nope, but I've always wanted one."

"Well, you're about to get four!"

"Oooo-kay," I said hesitantly.

Never having had a tattoo, I had zero understanding of how it felt, what it would look like or why I needed one in the first place. I had visions of angels with giant white wings encircled by barbed wire. Just then the nurse came at me with a marker, some sort of a sharp instrument and a tape measure. She measured across my chest width-wise and then horizontally down to my sternum area. She put four dots on me with the marker. Three of them were in a line horizontally across the top of my chest and one down the middle, resembling a "T" in shape. "OK, this next part may hurt a little bit."

"Bone marrow biopsies hurt! This should be just fine." My comments were as much to soothe my own worries as to let her know she wasn't going to hurt me.

She placed the sharp instrument on the top of the first marker dot and pressed hard. It was all I could do not to wince and let out a "yip." I was surprised at how much it actually did hurt. "You OK," she asked out of habit.

"Doing fine, but I'm not sure I want that life-sized tatt of an M1 Tank on my back anymore."

Both the nurse and assistant laughed out loud, just a bit louder than they thought they would. I felt another bead of sweat rolling down my armpit. "OK, let's finish these up and get you out of here, eh?"

"Sounds great."

Three more sharp pokes and my day was finished with these ladies. I sat up from the table, put my T-shirt back on and walked out, trying not to look at the embarrassingly sweat-soaked crinkle paper still left on the table.

The next morning I went into the radiation clinic and signed in. They had an outer waiting area and a smaller, inner waiting area. Not a good sign, right? But I was really surprised when the receptionist gave me a pager after I signed it at the outer desk.

"What's this for," I asked her.

"You can feel free to roam around the hospital and grounds. We'll page you when we're ready for you to go to the back."

I thought that was very cool. I took my pager and wandered off to the Starbuck's down the hall. Yes, Beaumont Hospital is that big. ;) I barely had my Grande, Soy, 150-degree Latte when my pager went off. *Here we go.*

I went back to the smaller waiting room and flipped through a couple of seriously outdated magazines on the table while I enjoyed my latte. I thought to myself, '*I probably shouldn't be touching these. You know how many other people have had their disgusting hands on these magazines? You know how many people don't wash their hands after using the bathroom? You know how often these magazines get washed?*' The time I spent without an immune system after my stem cell transplant changed how I viewed the world a bit. But before I could make it too far down my OCD path, the nurse's assistant came to the door of the waiting room.

"Donald Wilhelm," she inquired.

"Yep," I said as I stood up and I followed her back to the treatment area.

"OK, Donald, I need you to take off your shirt and lie down on the table." As I humbly obliged her request, I made sure my backne was not visible to the majority of the people present. I was so embarrassed of it that removing my shirt was literally the worst part of this entire ordeal. I started sweating....again.

I lay down on the treatment table covered in white crinkle paper. I felt the sweat beads rolling from my armpit down my upper ribs, around to my back and finally soaking into the crinkle paper. The nurse walked over to a shelf that housed all of the patient masks, retrieved my mask, and brought it over to me. It still reminded me of something we made in kindergarten. She walked over and placed it over my face.

"OK, Donald, I need you to relax and remain perfectly still OK?"

"Sure thing," I said.

This time, after she placed the mask on my face, she connected the two clips on either side of it to the table and clamped them down. I liken them to the clamps on a glass, airtight storage jar or the lid on a bottle of Grolsch beer, or the clasp on a metal toolbox. When she pressed the handles of the clamps down, the mask dug down into my forehead, the bridge of my nose, cheeks and my chin. I was paralyzed. I couldn't move my head even a slight bit. I had a momentary chill come over me. *Wow, I thought. This must be serious business. They're not taking any chances of me moving.*

As I lay on the table I looked above me at the massive "lens" of the radiation machine. Have you ever seen a movie about life on a submarine? You remember what the periscope looks like that the captain uses to see above water? Well that's what the radiation machine reminded me of. The nurse used some buttons and the big periscope lowered over my upper chest. The bottom of it was made of glass, so I could see up into it, but could never really make out what I was looking at. It had an elaborate maze of mirrors and lights that didn't seem to lead anywhere. The nurse continued to play with the buttons on the table until she was positive that the periscope lined up with the "T-shaped" tattoos she had placed on my chest previously. Now I understood how this whole thing works. My anxiety continued to build, and sweat continued to slip down my ribs and back.

"OK, Donald, we're ready to start. You OK?"

"Good as I'm gonna get," I mumbled with locked jaw.

"OK, we're gonna go into the control room now. There's microphones in here and a speaker so if you need anything just speak up and we'll be able to hear you."

"OK," I said. I had already learned through my medical-testing experience that "control room" was a euphemism for a safe place that the staff can hide to avoid whatever's about to come, point-blank out of the machine, aimed at my chest.

The machine switched on and ran for about three minutes. It was completely painless. I just wished I could have seen something recognizable in the labyrinth inside of the periscope. "OK, Donald…that's it," said the nurse as she stepped back into the treatment area.

"Seriously? That was no big deal."

I was elated by how easy radiation appeared. As I sat up from the treatment table, I snuck a look back at the crinkle paper on the exam table. It was soaked through, all the way across. I was so embarrassed that I just put my shirt on and made a B-line for the door.

Three weeks came and went in the radiation center, every day the same. Back in Dr. Jeff's office, my test results were back. The chemo and radiation had done their respective jobs. I was in remission again. As much as that word was meant to be a promise for the future, I had learned that it can be as empty as the smile on Dr. Jeff's face when he said it. Neither of us believed anymore. I had gone so far as to rename this period of time. I no longer called it "remission," but rather "intermission." The term refers to a short period of rest, prior to the next phase that is guaranteed to follow. It seemed to fit my situation better. I faked optimism on the outside as usual, but inside, I was exhausted from fighting this disease and from fighting my own thoughts. I just couldn't do this anymore on my own, I knew I needed help.

CHAPTER 15
Seeking Mental Help

What is it like to live with chronic anxiety? The term gets thrown around in everyday life now. Trust me, if you don't like sitting in rush hour traffic, or you're nervous about your job, that's not the kind of anxiety we're talking about here. This is where your thoughts of fear, doubt and self-consciousness are constant. Every 10 seconds, something would remind me of my cancer, causing a constricting in my chest and a hollow feeling in my stomach. I want you to think about that for a bit. I'm not joking when I say every 10 seconds. Imagine every constructive, fun or intimate thought process you have, being interrupted every 10 seconds with a message that says, "Your cancer is spreading, you're going to die." You try to push past the thoughts and get back to where you were, but you can only ever be semi-present in anything else.

All day, every day, 50% of my brain was running a self-destructive program that caused me mental distress as well as physical drain. At night, I would have headaches from over-thinking during the day. And the problem with the negative thinking was that it would happen so quickly I didn't even realize I was doing it. In Dr. Phil's book, *Self Matters*, which I cannot recommend strongly enough for every living person, he refers to these lightning fast, negative thoughts, as "tapes." They are self-defeating thoughts that are so over-learned that they run on autopilot, completely undetected, below the surface of your awareness. But the dangerous part about them is that they don't just interrupt your mental processes. They have a physiological impact on your body as well. In my case, uncontrolled sweating, backne, a tightening in the chest, a pit in my stomach, fatigue, daily heartburn and migraine headaches. All things I'd never had before my cancer. And the biggest impact of all, my internal stress was weakening my immune system and leaving me vulnerable. My fearful thoughts of the cancer regaining strength had become a self-fulfilling prophecy. The truly terrifying part: I knew all of this, but I still couldn't stop the "tapes." I knew in my heart that my negative thinking was the catalyst for my cancer. Dr. Phil sums it up succinctly: "The health professionals who treat you may have greater knowledge about your disease, but you have greater knowledge about you. Over the long haul, you have more power over your body and mind than anyone else. And you have more of the responsibility." I badly needed to get my power back.

I scheduled an appointment with a psychologist to talk about my anxiety. I had never done this before, and it can be quite intimidating. They ask you for a bunch of information over the phone, including the reason you're making the appointment. It's quite unnerving to admit to a strange voice over the phone that you have a mental problem. *I hope I'm not on speaker-phone. Does she write what I'm saying in my chart? Are they all going to look at me strangely and talk amongst themselves when I check in?*

I wanted to find a psychologist who was also a cancer survivor. I didn't then, nor do I now, believe that a mental healer can purport to give life advice to someone who's been through cancer if they haven't been there themselves. Ultimately, I just wanted someone to listen to me and understand what I had been through. I had been fighting this killer for four years now, on my own, and my soul longed to talk to someone who truly understood the burden I carried.

Alas, I could not find a doctor in all of metro Detroit that met this qualification. I settled on a woman who specialized in treating cancer patients, but was not herself a cancer survivor. I hoped that perhaps she may have a special insight that she gained from her years of interactions with patients like me.

We progressed through several appointments where we would take turns talking to one another. But we quickly reached a point when I started to feel frustrated. I felt like I wasn't getting to talk enough. All I really wanted was to spend my 50 minutes talking about what I'd been through. All I wanted from her was an occasional, "That must have been incredibly difficult for you. How did that make you feel?" But she couldn't see it. She wanted to focus on curing my anxiety, but we hadn't gotten to the core of why it was there in the first place. That's what I mean about having a counselor who has been where you've been. If she had been, she might have suggested that I book back-to-back-to-back appointments and just let me talk for three hours, mostly uninterrupted. I would have paid for that out of my pocket if my insurance wouldn't cover it.

I had, and still have, a lot of emotional burdens that I carry around from everything I've been through. Friends and family ask how you're doing, but they are just not an outlet that you can fully dump everything on. They need you to be strong, or at least look like it, because they're falling apart inside as well. After four years of treatment, I had been through so many experiences, most of them bad and most of them alone, that it would take me months to explain them to someone. But without the chance to talk about it all, you can't release it. It smolders in you and flares up on a breezy day when your guard is down. But in my case, it was like living in a wind tunnel, because the fire never waned. After several more appointments with my therapist, I realized I was going to have to do this on my own, like everything else. "You need to change the way you're thinking," she'd say to me.

No kidding. Isn't that what I'm paying you for? I thought in my most sarcastic scoff.

I'm sorry to say my takeaway from therapy was not a good one. I felt that my psychologist was well equipped to help her patients <u>identify</u> the problem of their negative thinking. But there really appeared to be no magic pill or technique on how to <u>fix</u> the problem. I had walked into the office on day one already aware of what I was doing wrong. What I needed was a regimen to fix the problem. Without a concrete solution, I struggled to stay focused on effecting real change.

During my third "intermission," I had begun to make some positive changes in my external life. I focused on hanging out with the few friends that I had left who were genuine people. Myself, Cousin Dave, Cousin Kevin and a few others, had barbeques together, rented movies, went on haunted hayrides and played cards. On the surface, I had begun to make the right choices on how to live my life. I was doing things that I did growing up. I played pick-up basketball, went rollerblading, fishing and camping. But during these fun activities, I still struggled at times with my nervous thoughts. I felt I was getting better, but not a rate that I wanted or needed to.

CHAPTER 16
Relapse #3

It was now late Fall of 2004 and time for my next checkup with Dr. Jeff. He ordered a CT scan so we could see what was happening inside of me. I had only been in remission for three months at this point.

Let me describe the CT testing process for those of you who have yet to have the pleasure. Let's say your test is on a Friday at 10 a.m. On Thursday afternoon, you'll need to swing into the hospital to pick up a quart of barium. This is a chemical substance in liquid form that makes your insides "light up" during the CT scan. It allows the radiologist to see your organs and also any abnormalities like tumors. They make the solution in several different flavors, but let me tell you right now, not a single one of them is tolerable. It's sort of like drinking liquid rubber or plastic, tainted with a slight hint of Tang or fruit punch. And its consistency is more slippery than wet.

First thing Friday morning, you'll need to make sure you finish the entire bottle before heading to the hospital for your scans. You'll gag, choke and maybe even tear up from this stuff, but somehow, you'll make it happen. You have to.

Feeling like the worst is over, you head into your appointment. You check in with the technician in the CT area. He or she will hand you a clipboard with the obligatory forms that always need to be filled out. You sign off saying you've read the privacy act, even though you barely glanced at the 3-page document printed in 10 font. After dutifully completing all of the forms, you hand them back and return to your chair. Now you need to decide if you'll read the 1 ½ year old golf magazines on the table in front of you, or watch the small television up in the corner that is broadcasting a morning talk show with its hosts taking turns trying to talk over one another on the topic of this year's hottest handbag designers. You decide to just close your eyes, lean your head back on the wall, and try to mentally block out the noise.

"Mr. Wilhelm," questions the tech, now standing next to you with a 32 oz Styrofoam cup in her outstretched right hand. You lift your head, open your eyes and instinctively reach out to take the cup from her.

"I need you to drink this entire cup of barium as fast as you can and then we can begin your scans."

"Outstanding," you sarcastically say. And you think to yourself, *maybe I should just eat the cup when I'm done as well.*

Five minutes later, after dismissing the temptation to pour half of your glass into the fake ficus plant next to you, you proudly announce to the tech that you're done.

"OK, come on back with me then," she says. She leads you past several small exam rooms and into the last room on the right side of the hall.

This is a fairly large room and outside of a couple chairs, the only thing in it is a huge machine in the center of the room. The machine resembles a giant white doughnut, with square edges and a small exam table on the front of it. "I need you to remove any metal you may have on because it will distort the CT images." So off comes your belt and watch. Now you lie down on the exam table and slide under the sheet that was laying over it. "I'll need you to undo your pants and slide them down to your knees. The metal in the zipper needs to be out of the CT range too." Feeling a little out of place now, you lie back and put your head onto the pocket-sized pillow she provided. The tech lifts your legs from underneath the sheet and slides a huge wedge-shaped pillow under your knees to make your back more comfortable.

"OK, I need to hook up an IV now. Is one arm better than the other?"

"Yes, my left one. In fact, just this one vein. All the rest are blown out by the chemo." You point to the small vein in the crook of your left arm, on the inside of your elbow. The tech places a tourniquet around your left bicep and begins to flick your vein. You absolutely hate when they flick at your veins. She swabs the spot with an alcohol pad and reaches for her needle. Success. And on the first time too.

Her instructions continue, "OK, I need you to put both of your arms straight back behind your head for the duration of the test. You can hold your left arm with your right, but don't move once we begin the testing. It's very important that you lie completely still for the whole test."

"No problem," you say, not having any idea how cramped your arms will be when the test is over in 10-15 minutes.

"Now we're going to run you through the machine a few times. The first one is for calibration. The machine will ask you to hold your breath at regular intervals. Then, I'm going to come back in and set up the machine to inject some iodine into your IV during the second pass. That provides a contrast on the films and allows us to see inside of you better. Any questions?"

"Nope," you say. "Let's get this show on the road."

As you lie on the table, the machine starts to whir behind you. It kind of sounds like a very quiet jet engine beginning to warm up. The exam table begins to inch you backwards into the donut hole. After alternately holding your breath and breathing deeply on command for about seven minutes, you open your eyes and find yourself on the opposite side of the doughnut hole. Next, the tech walks back into the room.

"OK," she said. "How you doing?"

"Fine."

"We're almost done. I'm going to set the machine to inject the iodine on this next pass. Now it's pushed in at a fast rate and that causes some people to have a *warm feeling* down below."

"Ohhhhh-kaaay," you say, still processing what the hell that statement is even supposed to mean.

The tech leaves the room and the table slowly begins to move. You hear a click from behind you and the machine releases the die into your IV. The first five seconds you're filled with comforting, almost Zen-like warmth throughout your whole body. It really is quite pleasant. But just then, you get this weird hot spot…, in your ass! It feels like you're losing control of your bowels and you instinctively clench your butt cheeks together as hard you can. A small panic sets in for another 10 seconds hoping your body doesn't do something to embarrass you. Finally, the feeling begins to fade. Without a doubt, it's one of the strangest things you'll experience along the cancer journey.

A few days later I was sitting in one of Dr. Jeff's exam rooms, waiting for my CT results. I was not confident. I was not hopeful. I wanted to be, but the little voice inside of me kept saying, *Nothing's changed. You still feel the same stress inside. You already know what the test says. Don't be naïve.*

I had learned to read Dr. Jeff's body signals upon entering the room. I could tell from the way he greeted me whether the test was good or bad. When he enters the room, he always smiles and says hello. He showed a good poker face at this point. But there is a direct correlation in the time it takes from him shaking my hand until he glances down at my chart. If the test was good, he chit chats longer and asks more personal questions about my life outside of cancer. If he has bad news to deliver, he is generally already looking towards my chart before we even finish the handshake…as he did on this visit.

"Well my friend, we've got some decisions to make. Your cancer is back. You've got tumors in your mid-chest, your abdomen, both shoulders and both sides of your neck. You also have a couple of small tumors on your liver, and you have an enlarged spleen."

I remained stoic, nodded my head and responded only with an "Hmmm."

He continued, "I think it's obvious that we need to try something more drastic. Your immune system, for whatever reason, is not able to kill your Hodgkin's. I think we should move onto another stem-cell transplant, this time using your brother Mike's cells. You have good odds that this can put you in remission again."

"Not sure about that, Dr. Jeff. I gotta do some more research and think this over. Can you just give me some information on what all's involved?"

Armed with the info on the recommended next steps, I went back to my apartment. I was unable to even contemplate the decision ahead of me. I sat there alone, staring out my sliding glass door looking into Bald Mountain State Park. It was a gorgeous view that I had enjoyed many times.

My second floor apartment backed up to thick hardwoods that regularly provided viewing of whitetail deer, foxes and dozens of different species of birds. There was a 20-foot tree that had been overtaken by Concord grape vines. The tree was still alive but the vines climbed right over the top of it. Not great for the tree's longevity, but the grapes were a particular favorite of the native birds, especially the cardinals. Each year, they would wait until winter had set in and the scene was blanketed with snow. For some reason, this triggered the cardinals' appetite for the grapes. They would come into that tree by the dozens. Only fifteen yards away, I would sit and watch them for as long as they stayed. Six inches tall, their bright red bodies decorated the tree from limb to limb. It was a living Christmas card, a bittersweet symphony that I didn't have the emotional capacity to enjoy right now. *Well, I've daydreamed long enough avoiding what's next! Get on with it, Son!*

I redoubled my research on Allogeneic stem cell transplants. It didn't take me very long at all to find the odds were not in my favor this go-round. A person who's had multiple relapses of Hodgkin's, by all accounts, had about a 40% chance of being cured by this treatment. And remember, the medical community considers the definition of "cured" to mean that you survive for an additional five years. Being in my early thirties, surviving five years was not much of a cure to me. In addition to the low cure rate, some researchers put my chance of dying from complications of the procedure between 25–35%! And that was the best case scenario, involving a donor who was a perfect match. Dejected, but feeling somewhat optionless now, I researched further. *All right, let's assume I survive this thing. What are the possible side effects outside of death?*

As I soon discovered, the list was long. Too long. Early complications could set in before I even left the hospital, during my **5-week stay**. Mouth sores and hair loss. I tried to stay open minded. *OK, no big deal, I've dealt with those already.*

Bleeding because of low red/white blood cells and platelets. *Well, I'll just have to be very careful and not cut myself. Guess it's electric razor only for a while.*

Nausea, vomiting, diarrhea. *Awe, they're old friends of mine at this point. No worries there.*

Depression and infertility. *Already got both of those...moving on.*

Infections, like shingles, herpes and pneumonia. *Ahhh, OK, that would suck!*

Cataracts, kidney, heart and/or lung disease. *Hmmmm...*

Recurrence of the same Hodgkin's Disease that the transplant was used to treat, and/or other cancers. *Christ, this is one piss-poor marketing message!*

Next, the long-term complications: Graft failure. The new stem cells don't work, or only work for a little while. Now I would have no immune system. *Wow, that would mean I'd have to be a bubble boy I guess...*

Graft-versus-host disease. (GVHD) The donated stem cells attack my body's own healthy cells and organs. This is because they recognize them as invaders. Once this sets in, it could take three years or more to resolve itself. It can affect the skin, the GI tract, the liver, or any other vital organ. Ultimately, it can lead to death. *Crap, we're right back at death again. I thought this was the non-lethal side-effect list???*

I spent a couple of weeks weighing my options. I was ping-ponging back and forth on an hourly basis. I needed to ponder the risk/reward ratio of the transplant procedure in its entirety.

CHAPTER 17
Parting Ways with Dr. Jeff

Dr. Jeff virtually burst into the exam room with my 6-inch thick medical file in his hand. He had a look of rekindled hope on his face. "You already know your brother Mike is a perfect stem cell match to you. Are we ready to get started?"

"Sort of," I said as I tried to feign excitement.

"I would say if we started on Monday getting the whole process going, we could schedule this transplant for a month from today."

Up to that last sentence, I had been intensely struggling with whether or not I was willing to undergo this transplant. As much as I respected Dr. Jeff and his knowledge, nothing we'd tried in the last 4+ years had made any difference. Now faced with another radical procedure, the voice inside of me that had been muted for years grabbed a bullhorn and started a protest rally. "This isn't necessary! You know what the problem is! You know how to heal yourself! Think rationally!"

I truly felt that I knew what needed to be done. I believed that my mostly negative emotions were at the core of my problem. Ground zero was my thought processes and the lack of personal happiness. I knew if I could improve what went on inside of me, I could build an environment that would allow my immune system to vanquish this houseguest from Hell. What I'd come to believe is that the constant anxiety surrounding treatment of my cancer was what kept empowering it. I needed to break the cycle. And I needed to do it without another transplant. "Dr. Jeff, I've made a decision. I'm making a colossal shift in how I approach my disease. At this time, I'm not willing to have the transplant." I watched as his shoulders slumped. I continued. "I think I can beat this thing on my own, based on what I've learned about my own body. I'm going to stop all treatments and work on getting myself genuinely happy.

I need to distance myself from all of this physical and mental torture. I think that's what my body needs in order to take over."

"You need to know, I give you about six months to live without any treatment." His comment was quiet and cautious.

I looked at Dr. Jeff intently so he knew that my decision had been cemented already. I could tell he was worried about me and thought that I was giving up. I tried to set his mind at ease. "If I'm wrong, Doc, I'm OK with that. I'll accept the consequences." We both stood up. He shook my hand and then put his arm around my shoulder. He opened the door and walked me out the front desk. This was his way of saying goodbye. We exchanged pleasantries, shook hands once more and I left the office. I would not return.

Now at this point, I feel it's imperative that I take a time out from my storyline and issue a warning. I came to my decision, fully armed with years of personal experience and research on my particular cancer and condition. Let me be painfully clear on this point: I am **not** encouraging, nor suggesting that anyone else choose to take the path I did. To this day, I believe in conventional medical treatment and insist that anyone reading my book trust in your doctor's wisdom. To borrow a powerful quote, "Do not substitute my judgment for your own." I learned some valuable lessons the hard way. Use what I've learned about the mental component of cancer in conjunction with conventional treatment. Go see a counselor, join a support group and follow you doctor's advice!

CHAPTER 18
On My Own

So there I was, early January of 2005. I was looking death in the face and issuing a challenge. The challenge was that death couldn't take me before I could live life to its fullest. But I had an advantage that death was unaware of. I was now measuring life, one present moment at a time. If the following Monday was a perfect day and then I died in my sleep, I would still have won. I stacked the odds of success and happiness in my favor and set out on my experiment.

After five years of near constant battle with my cancer, I began to stand-down from my warrior posture. My new approach was to take stock in what I could be thankful for. I began to appreciate everything in my life. I mean everything. If I had to park ½ mile away from the store or restaurant, I would think, *I'm so lucky to be alive and healthy enough to walk this distance. It's good exercise.* If a bird crapped on my car, I would think, *It's an amazing thing to be alive to witness bird poo. And besides, I like going through the car wash.*

I considered every moment to be a gift. And I filled all the space in my calendar that used to be consumed by cancer treatments with activities that I loved to do. I scheduled a ski trip with my Cousin Dave to Northern Michigan. I grew up on these ski hills, spending nearly every single winter afternoon on them as a high schooler. But somewhere along the line of adulthood, I let my passion for the sport slip away. It had been 10 years since I'd been skiing. I was embarrassed of myself for not putting myself and my likes ahead of other people's requests and demands. There, on the quad chair lift at Boyne Mountain Resort, I began to realize that I had a major self-esteem issue that needed to be resolved. My whole life, I had put other people's wants/needs above my own in an effort to gain their affection and approval. And what did that teach them? It taught them that my needs weren't that important. That if they pressed me, I would waffle and give in to them. Somewhere along the line, I associated other people's approval with personal happiness. What a hollow existence. This had to stop.

After my ski trip with Dave, I went out and purchased a snowmobile. I'd never been allowed to have one as a kid because my father hated them. He had valid reasons since trespassers would ride on our property and destroy small trees and plants that were partially hidden under the snow. But legal, respectful snowmobiling is done on groomed trails with laws and rules of the road. In fact, most trails are patrolled by local sheriff departments or Department of Natural Resources officers.

Snowmobiling quickly became a leading passion of mine. For me, it's the perfect pastime in the winter. It gets you out so you can enjoy nature. Many times I would ride the trail until I came to a secluded area. The pine trees were thick on either side of the trail. They reached from both sides over the top of the trail, forming a soft, evergreen tunnel. The fresh powdery snow covered the trees. I would pull my sled over to the right side of the trail and shut off the engine. I'd take off my helmet and just sit and listen. At times, the quiet could be deafening. And then, off to the right, I'd hear a squirrel rustling as he worked diligently to uncover some of the treasures he had buried last fall. And always the Chickadees would play in the branches. They would flutter from branch to branch, seemingly elated just to be alive. "Haaaaaaaaahhhhh." A long slow exhale and I would let a small piece of my cancer past go. If only for a few fleeting moments, this was a place to feel safe. To feel normal. To be whom I wanted to be.

Winter of 2005 slowly gave way to Spring in my home state of Michigan. Nature began to wake from its hibernation and with a host of new outdoor activities, drew me out of my apartment. Bald Mountain State Park, right outside my window, has an extensive trail system for hiking. One of the loops is almost five miles long, through thick forest. It has significant elevation changes and crosses streams and open fields. I found it very easy to forget that I lived in the Detroit metro area while hiking these trails. I would take time every day to hike the five mile loop. I walked briskly, completing the hike on average in 90 minutes. Though I often stopped along the way to reflect and enjoy nature. One day I would stop to listen to a loon on the inland lake next to the trail. Another, I would watch a jackrabbit as he sat and watched me. I never ignored a chance to appreciate my surroundings and contemplate my role in them.

During these times, my cancer became just a little more distant. It would fade just a tiny bit more with each excursion. Although it was still painfully prominent in my thoughts, I was gaining a sliver of control, one day at a time. Sure I would have loved the gratification of instantly forgetting everything about the last five years, but that's just not realistic. For those of you who are supporting someone with cancer, understand that even when they reach "remission" you can't expect them to snap back to the same person they were prior to diagnosis. They are irrevocably changed. The sounds, smells and pictures in their minds will blur at the edges over time, but they will never disappear. Support them. Ask questions. Listen for long periods of time. Don't give advice. Smile and tell jokes. Guess what? You're not the same person anymore either. Cancer changes everyone it touches. That's the silver lining of this disease.

CHAPTER 19
Remarkable Chain of Events

Summer was now in full effect. A remarkable chain of events was about to unfold that would take me to a place in life I couldn't believe.

One day, Cousin Dave called me up. "Hey Bro, guess what Kim and I just bought?"

"No clue Dave..., a new house?"

"Sort of. It has a bed, kitchen area and a bathroom. Except the bathroom is called a head."

"Dude!? You guys bought a boat?"

"Yup."

"Sweeeet! What kind?"

"It's an old '76 Chris Craft, 25ft overall."

"Rock on, Dave! When are we going for a boat ride?"

"Well, we were thinking of tonight. We were hoping you could join us since you grew up around boats and might be able to help us with a few things."

"I am there! Send me an email with directions, eh? Dude, this is totally awesome!"

Now for those of you that have never been to Southeast Michigan or closely studied a map of the area, you might not even recognize that there is a very large lake that separates us from Canada. It's called Lake St. Clair. It's not officially one of the "Great Lakes," but it's pretty damn big in its own right. It's about

26 miles long and 24 miles wide. This is where Detroit metro boaters keep their boats and spend most of their time during the summer months. Like most of the "transplants" that moved to Detroit, I pretty much had no idea what went on out on this lake. I had never been out there and never spent much time in that area, known as "The East Side."

Dave and Kim took me out on the lake for a lovely summer evening cruise. I gave Dave some generic tips for driving and docking the boat, and he taught me about some of the features of a boat this size. I grew up around boats, but small ones. Nothing over 19 feet. Nothing with a "down below." With Dave's boat safely docked back in his well, the three of us toasted their new purchase. "This is the coolest thing ever, guys. You understand I'm applying for the open deckhand position, right? Here's to the *Pescatore!* May she run steady and true."

Having no insight into the catalyst role that the *Pescatore* had begun in my life, I returned to my normal routine. I spent the days of June working, hiking, golfing and playing volleyball. One day, Cousin Dave calls me up with a strange new invitation. "Kim and I are going to Jobbie Nooner this Friday, you wanna go?"

"Isn't that a huge boat party out on Gull Island? I saw a special about it on Access Hollywood one time, but never been there."

"Me neither," says Dave. "But Kim says you have to see it to believe it."

"Let's do it."

"Cool, meet us at the boat at 10 a.m."

"In the morning?!? When does this party start?"

"The night before for a lot of people. It's out of control!"

"Sweet! I'll be there, Holmes."

Now depending on where you live in the world you may not have heard of Jobbie Nooner before. But believe me, it's an epic party that rivals anything you'll see in any of the major U.S. cities. Party-goers come from around the world now to be at this event. Imagine a small island; say the length of a football field, and twice the width. There's nothing on the island except tall grasses and large clumps of trees in the middle. Now try to imagine concentric circles of a thousand boats moored around this island. People are partying on the boats and walking around the island. Some folks are dressed for Marti Gras with crazy costumes on, others just their bathing suits, still others nothing at all. There are D.J.'s spinning the latest techno music and hot dog vendors cashing in on the rookies that forget to bring food to an all-day party. Simply epic. Don't take my word for it though. Go to www.jobbienooner.com and look at the pictures for yourself. *Except for you, Mom; any of my elder relatives; or my mother-in-law.* Simply Epic. :)

The week after Jobbie Nooner, I called Dave at work. "Hey man, what is your well number again?"

"B47, why?"

"Oh, cause I know the guy who just put his new boat into B44, across the dock from you."

"Cool, the more the merrier. Anyone I know?"

"You're talkin to him, Captain," I boasted with an implied 'tadow!!!' at the end of my sentence.

"What??!!?? You bought a boat? In a week? You're fucking crazy. What kind did you get?"

"It's a 27-foot Rinker...express cruiser. It's got a fore and aft cabin, full head with shower, galley with stove, sink, fridge and microwave."

"Nice! Well it looks like our alcohol bill for this summer just went up exponentially."

"Hahaha! No doubt. Gas bill too. You coming down to the marina tonight?"

"Yeah, Kim and I will be there around 6 p.m."

"All right, see you then. Don't stop for beer, my boat's already loaded down."

The funny thing about my impulse purchase of my boat was that I didn't have a single bit of buyer's remorse. That's highly unusual for me. I had spent hours online researching the boat I was considering. I hired a marine surveyor to inspect it, as well as a mechanic. The boat was in great shape and the price was right. The seller had purchased a bigger boat and needed to unload this one. Having two boat payments is a motivating factor to sell like no other. But the most assuring feelings I had came from some voice inside of me that said, "Your new place is on the water. You need this boat. Don't look back." So I didn't.

CHAPTER 20
Finally Ever After

Unbeknown to me, purchasing my boat was just another link in a chain of events that would take me to the happiest place of my life. You see, I had owned the boat for only a week. Although I lived in Lake Orion, Michigan, at the time, some 40 miles northwest of where I kept the boat on Lake St. Clair, I was spending more time in St. Clair Shores, Michigan. I was frequenting the restaurants and bars, trying to get to know the locals who all seemed to be part of this inviting boating community I had just bought my way into. On a random Tuesday evening, my friend Jay and I went to a bar/restaurant on the water called Jack's. In the summer they sponsor Tiki Tuesday every week. Their specialty: live music outdoors on their patio, big crowds and over-priced drinks. We were meeting up with Cousin Dave, Kim and some of her friends.

We had just finished dinner when I spotted two blonde women walking into a covered portion of the restaurant. I think Jay noticed me noticing them, and played his small part in the continuing domino effect. I quickly returned to the conversation at our table. I was not here to meet women. After all, I still had cancer; I just bought a boat; it was time to play a while for me. Well, about 10 minutes later, I look up and Jay had wandered over to where the two blonde women were sitting. They had a big table, enough to seat eight people. "Excuse me, ladies. Are you using the whole table, or could my friend and I use the last two seats on the end?"

"Sure, you can join us," said the taller blonde.

Her name was Amy and we spent the night talking about everything imaginable. Not stupid, fruitless conversations, but meaningful stuff. At one point she asked me, "What do you consider your greatest accomplishment in life?"

In a flash I knew the answer, but should I give it? I decided that if my health concerns were something that would prevent this potential relationship from growing, so be it. I was going to be open and honest, almost to a fault with this woman, and if she could handle what I was about to say, then rock on! "I'm a cancer survivor," I proudly exclaimed. Turns out, so was her mother. Now I'm not saying she didn't have a little voice inside her head that warned her to be careful and go slow, because she did. But she continued on, risking emotional snaring.

Six months later, after we had both fallen for each other, we were at a restaurant and I had asked her a question that had been weighing on my mind. We sat at a crowded outdoor patio, but in my mind we were the only two there. "I've had other women refuse to get close to me because they're worried I'm going to die early and they don't want to get hurt. Do you think you feel that way a little?" Amy pushed aside our sushi dishes, reached across the table and held my hands. "I love you today." She paused, allowing me time to ingest her words. "It won't hurt less to lose you now than it would later." Wow! I was blown away. This woman was completely in love with me and fully dedicated to "us" no matter what happened. I had never experienced that before. In an instant, I recognized all the relationship mistakes I had made in the past. What a stark difference.

If you are single and living with cancer, I'm going to point out something that most people don't talk about, but it's real. In today's society, you're damaged goods. Most healthy people have a hard time letting themselves get close to a cancer survivor. I understand why, and I'm sure if you think about it rationally, you do too. Most of the media coverage in this country is about the death toll that cancer inflicts each year. How many stories do you see about those of us who kick its ass? Not nearly enough. This country is terrified of cancer, and I don't believe that it should be. Of course I know it's a serious disease that can and does kill many. But in my battle, I found that controlling and improving my thoughts, attitudes and energies each day was the way to beat the monster. By turning my thoughts positive and really believing that my body was healing itself, my immune system took over and did its job. So you're single with cancer, huh? So what?!? Get yourself to a place in life where you're the happiest, at any cost. Love yourself. Get a little selfish and put your wants, needs and desires above all else. Maybe it's boating, skiing, mountain climbing, painting, writing, or teaching. When you meet a new person you're interested in, they will be drawn to your happiness. And stand confident and proud that you've been able to face down one of the most feared diseases of our time.

My relationship with Amy was, and still is to this day, amazing. We spent nearly all of our time together, learning everything about each other. Our dislikes and likes were totally in sync. Mayo instead of Miracle Whip; toilet paper over instead of under; no olives under any circumstance; all mushrooms- all the time.

As we grew closer, life and the future started to take on a resurrected meaning to me. I believe that there's an emotional side effect to cancer that becomes more prominent the longer you have it. You lose your belief that you have a long future ahead of you. Maybe it was because I read too much medical research on my disease over the years. That info all tends to be very cold and very bleak. I believe the reason I partied so hard and spent so much money was that I didn't care about the future. I didn't believe there would be one so what difference did it make? Falling in love with Amy helped reverse that. We happily made future plans together and began enacting them right after we got married. (Notice how I skipped way ahead there? Yeah, she said "Yes!") :)

We started a program to pay down our combined debts. We also started a little investment company. It's called F.E.A. Investments. It stands for "Finally Ever After." It's a phrase we came up with to describe our marriage. Since both of us had been married previously, it seemed like a perfect caption. It took more than 34 years for us to find each other and we each took some wrong turns on the way. But in the end, it all goes into making us who we are, so it was worth the wait in our eyes.

So F.E.A. Investments purchased a rental house in Roseville, Michigan, and then another in Gaylord, Michigan. Both of us had always dreamed of having a place in Northern Michigan we could vacation in, and now we had it. We were making our combined dreams come true on a daily basis. Another mental side effect, this time positive, of having cancer is that when you set your future goals, you tend to make them a reality much sooner than a normal person. Most people talk about their goals like the Tooth Fairy is supposed to deliver them or something. Please! This life rewards __action__. If you want something, *you* have to make it happen. Now is the time!!

The domino effect continued. The next thing I did was to cut ties with some people that I frequently socialized with that were holding me back emotion- ally. They were the type of people that seemed to care only about themselves.

And, unfortunately, I had been the type of person who was too willing to make excuses for them, rather than hold them accountable for their actions. Well no more! You are who you hang out with, or at least that's how the old saying goes. I was redefining my life, and I was only willing to accept positive additions to it. If you were negative, you were out.

Each day, I worked very hard to control my anxiety and fear about my cancer. I tried to learn how to replace negative thought patterns with positive ones. Sounds easy, I know. But if you don't already know the true undertaking that this really is, you most likely soon will.

CHAPTER 21
This Time's a Charm is Born

The more I looked towards my future, the brighter each day became. People would often comment on how amazing my positive attitude was and how contagious they found it. And after I explained about having cancer four times in five years, they would all say the same thing. "You should write a book!!"

"You think?"

"Totally. It's unbelievable what you've been through. You've literally seen and done it all."

"Yeah, I guess you're right. To me, it just seems normal."

What I came to realize was that I had lost my "normal person" objectivity as it relates to cancer. The battle that I had gone through was my reality. It didn't seem like that big of a deal because I didn't have any choice but to live it. I couldn't relate to how a normal person viewed it anymore. But thankfully, the more people that told me I should write a book, the more I began to regain this insight.

So at some point, I threw down the gauntlet and, with Amy's total support, began to write my story. I wanted to give cancer patients, survivors, caregivers, family members, friends and the world at large, a look into my experiences. I wanted them to be able to approach cancer armed with my enlightened viewpoint. Now I don't believe that anyone can live through another's experiences. I think that each of us is merely a sum total of our own experiences. But I hoped that my story could help open their eyes to be on the lookout for their own experiences that would follow. They needed to expect emotional growth from their time with cancer. They needed to know that cancer was not a death sentence. They needed to hear my story, told from the patient's perspective, loaded with the emotions that most books don't reveal.

Now I'm not saying all of my experiences were positive. Most of them down-right blew! But I learned a ton about life and myself along the way. I met some amazing people too. Cancer changed me forever. And for the better. Did you happen to see Ted Koppel's "Living with Cancer" on the Discovery Channel in 2007? Google it, I think it's still on YouTube. One of the statements that struck me the most was from Lance Armstrong. He was referencing his battle with cancer. He explained that he considered his cancer to be his #1 advantage over the greatest cyclists in the world. Through his treatments, he felt that he'd learned what true suffering was, which his competitors could not draw upon. He went on to add that his battle with cancer was more suffering **and** triumph than all seven of his wins at the Tour De France *combined*!!! My own personal example pales in comparison, but I think you get my point. As soon as possible, you need to get your head straight. You need to adopt a positive mental attitude and YOU are the only one that needs to believe in it. As the great mind, Charles Haanel, said, "You are your only patient." You can't fake it to yourself. It won't work. It took me 5 years to learn that lesson.

As I near the end of my cancer story, let me summarize the journey to this point:

1) Sinus Surgery
2) Lymph node biopsy surgery
3) Bone Marrow biopsy procedure
4) Six-months of Chemotherapy
5) Remission
6) Relapse
7) Lymph node biopsy surgery
8) Bone Marrow biopsy procedure
9) Autologous Stem Cell Transplant
   a) Stem cell harvesting
   b) Mega-dose, 24-hour chemo for a week
   c) Transplant ward
   d) Reinjection of harvested stem cells
   e) One month of isolation due to lack of immune system
10) Remission
11) Relapse
12) Bone Marrow biopsy procedure
13) Six-months of Chemotherapy combined with

14) Radiation therapy
15) Remission
16) Relapse
  a) Oncologist tells me he can't help me...'You're going to die...get your affairs in order...I'll try to keep you alive as long as I can, maybe six months.'
  b) Stopped all medical treatment and began living life just for me
17) Got happy.
18) Bought a snowmobile. Bought a boat.
19) Met Amy. Got even happier!

Five years of my life, summed up in sixteen bullet points. Even as I write this I'm overcome by the gravity of that list. I wonder if when I was first diagnosed, someone had shared the first 16 bullet points on that list with me, would I be here to write this story? Frightening thought. I'd like to believe that I would be.

Six months after ending all medical treatments, I scheduled a CT scan for an update. If my cancer had spread aggressively in that timeframe, Dr. Jeff and I agreed that we would begin chemo again to prolong my life as much as feasible.

By now, I had become a pro at getting CT's done. I always went to the same place, with the same people working there. I walked in for my appointment in a t-shirt, cargo shorts and flip flops, the standard outfit for a boater in Michigan. Because of my time in the sun, I was quite tan as you would guess. I approached the CT technician and he said, "Wow, you look healthier than I've ever seen you. And happier too."

"Thank you. I've learned to actually feel that way, not just look like I do."

We both laughed and he began the usual process of hooking me up to the IV.

Two days later, I pick up my results from the test. Most people don't get this option since the results are sent to their doctor confidentially. But given my rapport with the CT staff, they knew I wanted to know results as soon as they were available and that I had the "on-the-job-training" now to be able to interpret the report. I picked up the report and went out to my car. I sat in the driver's seat for a few moments, eyes closed, breathing deeply, clearing my mind. The report was in a large manila envelope held in both hands on my lap. After about three minutes, I bent the two metal flap holders of the envelope upwards and pulled out the contents. My eyes scanned the report's first page. Skipping past the first three paragraphs of medical yadda-yadda-yadda, I hit the meat of the report.

'Blah, blah, blah...*patient shows a marked reduction in tumor mass*...blah, blah, blah." A shiver started on the back of my scalp and rocketed down to my feet and back up. I started crying. I was getting better! I was winning, all on my own. I knew all along that this was the solution for me, but I was too afraid to try it in the face of all the bleak information I was getting from science. I sat in the parking lot, numb but joyous, for another five minutes before calmly starting my car and driving home.

It was only then that the gravity of my decision to abort medical treatment truly set in. I knew my theories about positive mental attitude were correct, but still, I can't believe I put everything to risk in order to test them. But now as I look back, I really believe that if you can't "go all in", to borrow a poker term, you can't expect to win most hands you're dealt. You've got to be able to evaluate the risk/reward ratio. If the potential payoff for the gamble far outweighs the risk of the possible loss, you have to act on it. In my case, I was given six months to live. So I was risking some portion of six months. Maybe it was six months, maybe it was only 1 month. But the potential reward, if I was right, was years and decades of the rest of my life.

CHAPTER 22
Some Humble Advice

You know how I look at cancer and, in fact, most problems that come up in life now? I use an analogy of Chinese finger cuffs. The more you pull and resist the problem, the tighter it seems to grip you. I may never really be "out of the woods" when it comes to my health. But I'm OK with that. I consider every day to be a blessing. I am a lucky man. My finger cuffs are off permanently.

First time's a charm?
Second time's a charm?
Third time's a charm?
THIS TIME'S A CHARM! Does it really matter how many times it takes to beat something like cancer? Someone once said, "There's two types of people; survivors and die-ers." While the summation is a bit callous, I believe there's some truth in the sentiment. "If you want to be a survivor, you best gits to livin!"

CHAPTER 23
C.U.R.E. (Cause You Are Energy)

Everything in the world is made of energy. It's the base component for all that exists. Further, energy attracts like energy. Additionally, we are the sum totals of our personal experiences. So if you are an optimistic person who enjoys learning from your experiences, you likely possess a very positive energy. The Universe, or God (your preference on what to call the Divine power) rewards positive energy with positive outcomes. The more you genuinely expect good results, the more good results you will see. Conversely, if you're someone who's had a rough go of it, and you carry your battle scars on your sleeves for everyone to pity, life probably seems cumbersome. The Universe is picking up the negative energy you are emitting and responding with more outcomes to pity you for.

I want you to listen to me right now. You know me well enough now that I feel I should be able to ask you for a favor. Finish reading this book. Get to your preferred book peddler. Purchase *The Secret,* by Rhonda Walker. Read it and change your life. Then email me at dwilhelm@thistimesacharm.com and let me know how it impacted you. I'm wagering that you'll thank me for the referral and realize in the end, that I was actually asking you to do yourself a favor.

CHAPTER 24
Closing Thoughts

Over my six years during and post cancer, many people have asked me for advice for loved ones recently diagnosed. I'm honored to be in a position to give them advice. To quote a Chinese Proverb: "To know the road ahead, ask those coming back." I'm going to end this book by giving you all of the advice that I have given others in hopes that you will apply it to your own situation.

I hope by this point in the book you realize that cancer is NOT a death sentence. It is not a medieval plague. In fact, did you know that a cancer cell is simply a normal cell that is immortal? It's true. All cells have a lifespan and are supposed to die off on schedule to retain the body's balance. But cancer cells never die, they just keep multiplying. They multiply until they get in the way of a normal organ or system.

Step One: Change the way you view your disease. Release the fear you're holding inside. Don't spend energy trying to understand why or how you got cancer. Focus on the task at hand, getting better. Spend time thinking about how incredible the anatomy of your body is. How complex of a machine you really are. Admire your own engineering.

Step Two: Believe that you have the power to heal yourself with the right positive attitude. Hippocrates, the father of modern medicine, explained that the body, specifically the mind, is its own pharmacy. He knew that patients had the power to heal themselves if they really believed they could. That's why graduating doctors today still take the Hippocratic oath. In a nutshell, doctors pledge: "Above all else, do no harm." Hippocrates wanted to make sure that the medical intervention doctors give never interferes with the patient's own ability to cure himself. That's a powerful philosophy that I believe has been lost in today's modern medicine.

Step Three: Do your own research about your disease. Don't just rely on what your doctors tell you. Some oncologists are excellent doctors who understand the mind/body connection and can act as your coach when you need someone to inspire you. But unfortunately, a lot of doctors have their heads down and spend their day mired in the statistics of your particular cancer. Said differently, you are your disease to them and they go about treating you the way they were taught to and never deviate. That's why you need to be an expert in your disease. At times you will be called upon to make very important decisions in your treatment process. Make an informed decision.

Step Four: Be willing to question authority. Doctors are human. They make mistakes. Some doctors are excellent. Some suck. I have met more than a couple of really lousy physicians in my life I'm sorry to say. They don't keep up with medical research and they don't like to be questioned. Tough shit! This is your life at stake here. You are in charge. The doctor is a player on your team. An important player, but not the owner. You are the owner. You know your body better than they do. Make sure you both realize that.

Step Five: Control any anxiety or stress you have. It's completely normal to have both when facing a challenge like cancer. But you have to keep them in check because they do not serve you. Stress and anxiety wear down your immune system and allow cancer cells to flourish. "What you're eating is not as important as what's eating you." – Dr. Patrick Quillin

Step Six: Make future plans and believe in them. You need to see yourself in the future, healthy and happy with your life. You need to set attainable goals and work towards them every day.

Step Seven: Eat right. Enough said.

Step Eight: Exercise. Cancer is anaerobic, which means it thrives in an environment low in oxygen. Regular exercise, 30 minutes of cardio five times a week, oxygenates your cells. It also strengthens your immune system and gives you a positive attitude towards your body.

Step Nine: Learn how to meditate and do it daily. It only takes 10 minutes a day once you learn how to do it. It rejuvenates you, mind and body. It's better than a nap. It soothes your soul.

Step Ten: Spend some time each week alone, doing what makes you the happiest. No one is guaranteed any specific amount of time in this world. Though you are facing a life-threatening illness, you may get killed in a car accident on the way to your chemo treatment. Or worse, on the way home from it. It's a grim thought, I know. But it's a fact. You need to enjoy your life starting today, not when the doctor says you're in remission. Start right now. Never stop.

Step Eleven: Be happy. Why would you choose to live any other way?

As you begin your contest with cancer, I'm going to leave you by giving a pre-game "pep talk." Vince Lombardi, legendary football coach, said, "It's not whether you get knocked down, but whether you get back up." I believe there's more wisdom in those words than most pieces of advice you'll come by. You <u>are</u> going to get knocked down. It's life. But see it for what it is, know that it's a normal process, and pick yourself back up. The more you move forward through trying times, the more you'll grow to appreciate those times when you're on the other side of them. They will change you for the better if you appreciate them. This is a "teaching life." Learn from your experiences. Live your life. Love those that deserve it. Write a book. ;)

www.ingramcontent.com/pod-product-compliance
Lightning Source LLC
Chambersburg PA
CBHW031213270326
41931CB00006B/544